HOSPITAL BATTLEFIELD

A FIELD MANUAL FOR SURVIVAL

Bedside Strategies to Protect
Patients from Medical Errors
and Hospital Infections

Lynne Golonka, Ed. D.
Joseph Golonka, M.D.

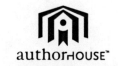

authorHOUSE™

1663 LIBERTY DRIVE, SUITE 200
BLOOMINGTON, INDIANA 47403
(800) 839-8640
WWW.AUTHORHOUSE.COM

First published by AuthorHouse 08/24/05

ISBN: 1-4208-7350-4 (sc)

Library of Congress Control Number: 2005907025

Printed in the United States of America
Bloomington, Indiana

This book is printed on acid-free paper.

Contents

Part One
Preparation for Battle

Part Two
Deployment

Part Three
Engagement

Part Four
Being Shipped Home

ACKNOWLEDGEMENTS

There are many individuals to thank. First, our Irish Setter, Mac, who didn't write a word, but kept us centered and sane. He's getting old, but aren't we all. Secondly, and more importantly, family, friends and professionals who generously supported us and acted as our first classroom for the book. Heartfelt thanks to the following readers, who asked the questions you, the final reader would have asked. Charlotte Carter, mediation colleague who asked "how, when and why" and kept us focused; Maureen O'Connell, RN, coronary care nurse who exemplifies the kind of nurse that we all want caring for us; Harriet, my sister and friend, who had recent personal involvement with hospitals; Susan and Don Cohen, long-time friends who also have experienced the health care system, more than they would have liked. Deb Prud'homme was more than our typist but also a friend. Everything arrived on time and freed us from the tyranny of Microsoft Word allowing us to think (a somewhat important part of writing). Thanks to Luke Santiago, graphic arts student who captured the spirit of the journey in his pen and ink drawings.

We also thank the hundreds of nursing students and medical residents who kept us on our toes at all times. We hope their professions are satisfying and they are giving the quality care we believe is the patient's right. A final thanks to the patients who helped us to grow both professionally and individually.

Last, but not least, our children, who as readers have finally proven useful. They had no trouble criticizing their parents, and are, to our delight, intelligent, loving, insightful adults.

WHY WE WROTE THE BOOK

The basic idea for this book came from discussions with fellow doctors and nurses. Many emphatically stated that they would avoid hospitalization at all costs. If it were absolutely necessary, they would use their knowledge of the system to protect their families and themselves. This book will allow you to share the insider's view of the system as well as prepare you to participate in the hospital experience, develop allies, and win the battle over illness.

Why do you need a battle plan? In one word: survival. Experts keep telling you to get information and ask questions. If you don't have an overall plan to use the information and develop strategies for survival, information is literally and figuratively a dead end. When do you ask the healthcare questions, and equally important, how do you ask the questions that can spell the difference between disaster and control of the situation? Who are those individuals who supervise and decide your fate in the hospital? What motivates them, how did they get there? How can you use the system to your advantage?

Hospitals and professional organizations cannot deny that serious medical errors occur and cause death. The 1999 study by the Institute of Medicine reported startling statistics. As many as 98,000 people will die in hospitals each year as a result. Plans are in place in many hospitals to lessen errors. Legislators are looking at bills to address the problem. All of this is positive, but will they work and how many lives will they actually save? In a May 2005, Journal of the American Medical Association article, it was reported that while improvements have been made, progress has been slow. In the interim, one does not wish to be a statistic at the hospital that did not initiate change. Actions taken in this area are a step forward but is it enough to protect you and your family in time? Systems change very slowly and we want to be proactive when it comes to our health and lives.

Real change comes from the grassroots, in this case at the bedside with the patient. Let the politicians, physicians, hospitals, lawyers, professional organizations, and insurance companies argue that health care needs help. While this is going on, assume control and take those actions that will insure survival and health. What we are calling for in this book is <u>vigilance and action at the bedside.</u>

This is not a professional book; it is a book written by professionals. If you're looking for a scholarly book with an impressive bibliography, numerous footnotes, and statistics, this is not for you. Put it down before you spend money on it. If you want practical advice from years of experience, we believe you'll find it here.

How the Book Was Written

When I've read a non-fiction book, particularly with co-authors, I always wondered who wrote what material: Whose voice am I hearing in written form? We could use the old "author one" and "author two" device, but that's confusing. A straightforward statement frees both the author and the reader and establishes honest communication.

Lynne wrote the first three parts with constant editing by Joseph for content, medical accuracy, and language, to be honest, more than I wanted. Joseph wrote Part Four with "ongoing, loving support" from Lynne. Actually, Lynne turned Part Four into a mediation format.

Each section is written in a different voice: counselor, teacher, nurse, mediator, and doctor. Don't get frightened, it isn't a case of multiple personalities, but rather multiple expertise, experience, and beliefs about quality heath care.

Part One: *Preparation for Battle* – Voices: Counselor and Nurse
Part Two: *Deployment* – Voices: Counselor and Teacher
Part Three: *Engagement* – Voices: Nurse and Doctor
Part Four: *Being Shipped Home* – Voices: Doctor and Mediator

One goal of this book is to take complex issues and present them in simple terms and to that end we have included editorial cartoons. Nothing seems to simplify life in a few strokes of a pen and one succinct line as they do. Every discussion needs humor and we hope you enjoy them. We certainly enjoyed choosing them.

The clinical tales of interactions are slices from our professional lives and are important illustrations of the core beliefs of the book, the absolute necessity for patients and families to have meaningful, knowledgeable interactions with those who care for them.

Our fifteen readers acted as a first semester class in Hospitalization 101 and their questions, criticisms, and suggestions served to keep us on target. This is our personal view of hospital health care with its strengths and weaknesses.

Lynne views this book as a realistic philosophical book or a philosophical realistic book, which is an oxymoron, a word she always wanted to use in conversation or writing. Joe views it as an opportunity to share knowledge and information. Both views of life have blended for the last forty-five years.

This book will not give you recommendations on illnesses, diagnosis, or treatments. Our goal is to help you understand the system through insider information and strategies. It certainly is not the opinion of all the health care agencies that employed us. In fact, they may prefer we didn't write this book. It is the pulling together of 40 years as a nurse, 30 years as a practicing physician, 22 years teaching nursing, 26 years as a therapist, 10 years as a mediator and 16 years as a consultant and medical director in a health insurance company. We believe you will find all those years have provided us with the knowledge that can help you win the most important battle of you or your family's life, hospitalization.

It is said that the best defense is a good offense. Let us teach you active strategies based on knowledge, skills and insight into the system. Attacking hospitals, doctors and nurses is ineffective and counter-productive to your battle with the real enemy, your illness. We began writing this book with the goal of not frightening the reader. Rather, our goal was to help you to take action through knowledge and skills. But in reality you should be scared. We are.

Dedicated to the Memory of Our Parents
Irene and Harry
Agnes and Emil

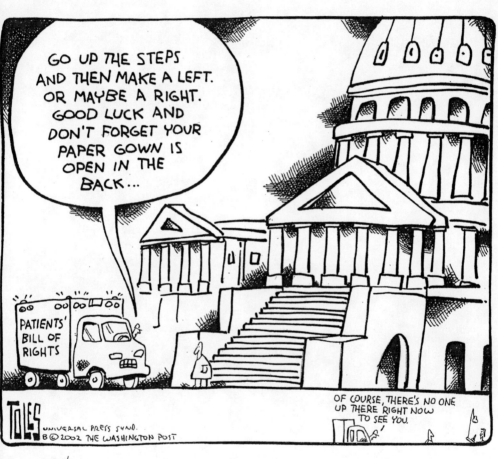

PART ONE

PREPARATION FOR BATTLE

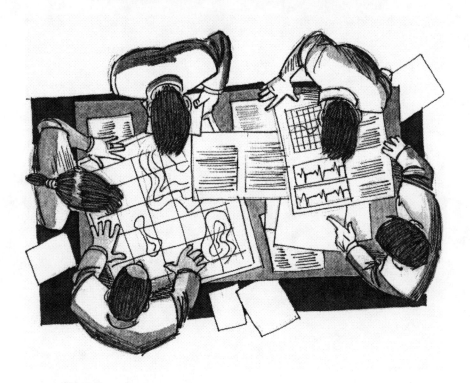

Voices:
Counselor and Nurse

CREATING A BATTLE PLAN

Gone are the days when preparation for hospitalization was planning what to bring with you, who would drive you there and bring you home and who would do your job or care for your family while you were in the hospital. It is now a matter of life and death.

The newspaper headlines are too frightening for that casual outlook. In the last two years the following headlines are a rallying call for action:

"Death Beds", *Chicago Tribune*

"Despite Efforts, Medical Errors Go On Killing", *The Washington Post*

"Nasty Germs Getting Even Nastier", *Associated Press*

"Basic Errors Plague Even Top Hospitals", *The New York Times*

"Study Finds High Rate of Drug Errors in Hospitals", *Associated Press*

"U.S. Survey Finds Medical Mistakes Common", *USA Today*

"Overworked Nurses Cited As Deadly Danger", *Associated Press*

You are literally in a battle for your life and you need to rally all of your resources - cognitive, emotional and communicative skills for success. Soldiers approaching a battle do it carefully, are well trained and are always fully aware of the great danger they face. Your battle plan for hospitalization acknowledges the danger, and in a preemptive strike, your intent is to take control. This plan needs to be developed before the actual engagement and can be viewed as an exercise in maximizing health and preventing illness. If your family enjoys computer games, view your battle plan as an interactive game with reality results. Armies often engage in war games.

If an unexpected hospitalization occurs through the emergency room, your battle plan is ready to implement. You have prepared yourself and your family to have more control over the situation. Safety experts advise families to have fire drill plans, including exit strategies. Each family needs a hospital plan with delegation of responsibility and pre-admission knowledge and skills.

Preliminary planning builds on three assessments:

1) Understanding of you and your family's strengths and weaknesses.

2) Clarity on who the enemy is with its strengths and weaknesses.

3) Recognition and utilization of allies.

The purpose of the battle plan is to weaken the enemy, the illness, and maximize and enhance your own strengths. The plan should be written, updated as new information is obtained, shared with all family members and specific about details, circumstances and personnel.

Visualize a war room as presented in movies and television. There are charts and graphs, models and games, telephones, computers and multiple soldiers and planners. Analysis of incoming data is a crucial component in this room. Let's turn your kitchen table, computer desk or family room into a planning site. This is serious, life-preserving business and the more focused you and your family become in planning and assessment, the more successful you will be.

Troop Assessment

Any battle plan includes an assessment of the troops. Are they prepared to contain and attack the enemy, illness? Have they been adequately trained? Do we have enough of them? You and your family members and friends are the troops. What strengths and weaknesses do you possess?

Let's start with weaknesses and strategize methodologies that will, at the very least contain them but more important change these weaknesses into strengths. At the end of each section, note pages are included to allow the reader and family to individualize their plan and list their own strengths and weaknesses. One identified weakness is lack of knowledge, and hand in hand with this knowledge deficit is the sheer complexity of what you need to know. The knowledge is in a foreign language, and just translating it can be an overwhelming task.

So often, articles and books advise the reader to ask questions. But how does one ask questions when you have no basic knowledge, beyond some generalities, you obtained from newspapers and the Web? You need to understand what you are asking so you can follow up with those crucial second and third questions. We've listed multiple questions, directed at specific procedures that you can use. You don't have to use the words in this book, but they are a jumping-off point for obtaining answers. Of key importance are the "what-if" questions. They are absolutely essential to successful questioning about your hospital care. We are speaking to the reader who will be a future patient or the family and friends of that future patient. Ideally, patients will be prepared to ask the questions and monitor their ongoing care themselves. Other patients may need their support team to assume this role. The "you" in the book refers to all of you who are waging this battle against illness. The active soldier will vary throughout the hospitalization. We are examining the deployment of troops in the most effective and life saving manner.

Another weakness is that you are ill. You are not at your strongest point in life. Therefore, your battle plan needs to be a team approach. Other individuals can balance the physical and emotional weakness that you more than likely will be experiencing at this time. A final weakness you experience comes from the intimidation factor of the hospital system itself. That big building on the hill is foreign territory, populated by health care workers in various roles and with different skill levels. In this book you will find strategies that can cut that intimidation factor down to a manageable size through insider information.

Every soldier needs to understand his strengths. Here are some strengths you may not realize you possess:

- Instinct for self-preservation
- Understanding of personal vulnerability
- Anxiety
- Anger
- Need for social support
- Planning ability

All of the above strengths are human responses and skills that we all possess. When facing a hospitalization for a family member or ourselves we need to bring them forth and use them. They are our ammunition in the battle against illness.

Self-Preservation

Your sense of self involves knowing who you are and the deep, ingrained desire to preserve that person against all attacks. This desire to live is extremely strong. Your desire to live unscathed is strong motivation to learn everything you can. Use this instinct to live as a catalyst to encourage you to become knowledgeable and skillful in your hospital battle against illness. Every soldier knows that his survival depends on learning as much as he can and developing skills for himself and his fellow soldiers in order to survive. In this book we have used the masculine pronoun for *soldier* in order to simplify the language. Of course, we're referring to all of the courageous soldiers of both genders.

Vulnerability

The ability to accurately express your vulnerability is an individual's greatest strength. Too many view this as a weakness when in reality only the strong can do this. The person who comes for counseling or seeks help is exhibiting amazing strengths. Pretending you are not vulnerable takes too much energy and puts you at a disadvantage. Every soldier knows and admits he is vulnerable to injury and death. The acknowledgment of vulnerability is the first step in self-preservation and continued vigilance.

A part of the reluctance to admit vulnerability is the equation that states to be vulnerable is to be helpless which is far from the truth. Let's look at definitions:

Vulnerable – Capable of being wounded; susceptible to wounds or injuries, literally or figuratively.

Helpless – Incapable of acting without assistance; needing help, incapable of self support or self defense, feeble.

You are not helpless!

"What can I do, I feel so helpless. I must stay in control at all costs. I'll show them, I'm not going to be dependent - I run my own company, take care of my family - no one's going to make me feel needy."

You have to realize that vulnerability can be your most effective defense. It is frightening to admit one is vulnerable but realistically, by recognizing this condition, you can use it to your advantage. Health care workers, by their very nature and training, respond positively to need. We use it in future questions to illustrate "I messages" that in a sense hook the caregiver into doing what they do best, give care. Seems logical, but the key is to accept your own vulnerability, not helplessness, but vulnerability.

You may find listing the emotions of anxiety and anger as strengths surprising. And because these two emotions are often viewed as negatives, we need to examine their contributions to the battle plan.

Hospital Anxiety

Every patient admitted to a hospital is anxious. The degree of anxiety is variable and is not necessarily tied to the severity of the illness. Some individuals face open heart surgery with calm while others are blown away by the thought of minor, elective surgery. Anxiety, in itself, is not a bad emotion as long as it is not allowed to get beyond your control. Any good soldier going into battle is anxious and this controlled anxiety helps to protect him. Senses are sharpened, learned skills are finely tuned, and he is always on the alert. No one wants to be fighting next to someone who really isn't as committed; then everyone in the unit is in danger.

Anxiety can help focus resources and provide the vigilance that can insure victory. It is only detrimental when you cannot focus on the battle, listen to the commands and take appropriate action. You need to channel your anxiety and use it as a tool to overcome the enemy. The knowledge and actions that are presented in this book will help to lessen anxiety and use it constructively. Verbalize it to professionals to increase support and as you take a more active role in your care, you will feel more in control.

Hospital Anger

Another emotion that one experiences during a hospitalization is anger. As with anxiety, this is an expected, normal emotional response. The healthy use of anger is to channel it into constructive life-preserving behavior. The final key to appropriate use of anger is to not displace it onto the nearest caregiver. You know the old example: the boss yells at his employee, John; John comes home, yells at his wife, Beth; Beth yells at her child, Tim; Tim yells at the dog, Gus; and Gus chases the cat, Tiger.

Your hospital anger needs to be directed toward the illness, not the nurse who is changing your dressing, or the doctor who arrives later than you expected or the wife who is checking to see how you are. Recognizing your anger is the first step in directing your anger energy toward healing.

In your planning, you will talk to other individuals, but don't let friends or relatives overwhelm you with their war stories. You don't have to fight their battles. I'm reminded of working as a mediator with couples going through a divorce. So often friends and relatives have their own marriage and gender wars and they then expect you to continue their battles and win the divorce war that they feel they've lost. If the advice and stories become overwhelming, just say, "It sounds like that was very difficult for you but hearing it makes me more anxious. Is there any one recommendation that you feel will help me?"

Fight your own battles, not the residual anger your aunt has toward her doctors or the resentment your friend feels toward one specific nurse. Keep the battle lines clear and focused, not their battle with the personnel. Be as single minded as you can in your fight against illness. Zero in on your target and use your energy to get well.

You are angry at being sick; this illness has changed your life and caused you pain. Focus your anger by taking a vague, generalized anger that is often displaced to personnel and give it a target - your enemy, illness. We look at anger, both patient and family, in more depth in *Psychological Warfare*.

Social Support

The need for social support of some kind is generally accepted in our society and is viewed in a positive light. How to best use this social support can pose a dilemma for patients and families. This social support needs to be systematically integrated into the battle plan by delegated responsibilities to friends and family through all stages of the battle.

I have interspersed clinical tales throughout the book. They could be called vignettes but that isn't my style. I thought of Chaucer and his Tales, journeys on the way to a destination. These have been a part of my clinical journey and I share them with you so you can journey with me.

Gypsy Family

Years ago in a local hospital, an elderly patriarch of a gypsy family was admitted in critical condition, near death. In those long ago days, families were considered incidental to the patient's recovery. However, based on their gypsy tradition and values, they insisted that the whole family, all thirty-five members, be present at all times for their loved one. They refused to move. The hospital did respond and all of the family found space in various waiting rooms, while three or four were at the bedside of their loved one on a rotating basis.

There was great wisdom in their insistence on being present. We're not suggesting that you have thirty-five team members, but the more allies you enlist in your battle, the more power you possess.

Every individual has his or her own sense of personal space, and the number of team members directly involved in your planning and hospitalization will vary from person to person. The members of the team can have various roles at different times in your plan. Our recommendation: Don't go it alone, the more team members the better. Some people are embarrassed to get sick and have to be hospitalized. "I'll just go in, have the operation done, get out and no one will know." Illness at some time happens to everyone and trying to hide it severely limits your options and ability to get help. Support and help translates to a successful battle against the illness.

Related to the need for social support is the individual's verbal ability to express needs. This is not always easy to do since it is related to our vulnerability. Recognition of our need for social support and verbally expressing needs to care givers and your support team can maximize your strengths to fight illness and ultimately win the battle. We recognize that there are different levels of comfort in expressing need. However, handling pain stoically or not telling caregivers about new symptoms can be deadly. Expression of emotional needs is difficult, but allowing yourself to say,

- *I'm scared.*
- *I'm really anxious about this operation.*
- *I'm edgy, I just feel so angry and I don't know why.*

can help you fight your illness.

Ability to Plan for Hospitalization

The final strength is your cognitive ability to learn basic skills needed for survival. Reading this book can give you a learning edge that can pull together all the strengths necessary to win the battle against illness. Examples of how to use these strengths will be illustrated throughout the book.

Some individuals love to plan; lists are used in day-to-day living. Others prefer to wait to see what happens. A basic concept of this book is that if you wait to have a hospital battle plan, it could be deadly. Soldiers don't wait to see what happens. They never lose sight of their enemy. You and your family need to be just as focused and use this book with its planning format as the structure of your own hospital fight against illness and complications. Now we proceed from your team to the enemy.

IDENTIFYING THE ENEMY

The big question of this section is "Who is your enemy?" It seems like a simple question but the key to winning a war is knowing your enemy totally so that surprises will be kept to a minimum. Your knowledge of the enemy can be used against him.

- How does he think?
- What are his resources?
- How has he fought in the past?
- Does he have allies?

Obviously, your illness enemy doesn't think but as medical science has shown, infections, bacteria and viruses in particular, have amazing adaptive powers. We have a record of how the illness has manifested itself in the past and its resources for multiplication and spread. You could argue that the illness' allies are other illnesses and infections that weaken the body and impair body defenses. The key ally of illness we will seek to conquer is hospital errors.

You can't have a battle plan unless you are completely clear on who your enemy is. Ask any soldier - if the enemy is clear, the battle plan can proceed. If the enemy is an insurgent, in civilian garb and hidden among civilians, the battle becomes more difficult and dangerous. Medical errors and hospital infections hide, then attack when you are most vulnerable.

What are his weaknesses? What are his strengths? How will he use the terrain? Absolute clarity and understanding of the enemy maximizes the potential for a successful war.

Illness Enemy

It seems self evident that the enemy is the illness but too often our focus and energy gets sidetracked to personnel, and the health care system in general. Zero in and visualize your enemy. Give the illness a name and a personality. Cancer patients are often encouraged to visualize the chemotherapy actually attacking and killing the cancer cells. If the illness and all of its manifestations are recognized and targeted, peripheral waste of energy will be minimized. No soldier in battle should focus on what's wrong with the army system, or those individuals he doesn't like.

Your enemy is the illness that has caused this hospitalization and the illnesses' allies can be defined as complications. Visualize your heart attack as the enemy and a concurrent, respiratory infection as the enemy's ally that weakens your body and can cause death.

Illness is a tough enemy because it changes its shape and weapons as the battle continues. Don't let your focus on the enemy get diffused and scattered onto personnel in the war zone. Focus on the enemy's strengths and weaknesses.

Enemy Strengths

The enemy, the illness, has in a sense become stronger since you now face hospitalization, and this fact will play a major role in whether you win or lose in your battle.

I'm going to the hospital to get better is now a naïve view of the situation. It's the outcome everyone wants and hopefully gets, but the outcome is not a sure thing. The hospital should be considered the site for your battle plan. It is one part of the plan that you can learn to monitor in order to allow it to become a true healing place. The strength of the enemy is at this time overwhelming. The illness has the upper hand and it requires hospitalization. It has overwhelmed your resources and put you in a defensive position. The very complexity of the illness and the multiple symptoms make it a formidable foe. The illness has affected you anatomically and physiologically. Not only is your structure under attack, but each of your body systems and their functions are vulnerable. What affects one part of your body affects the whole organism.

This illness also has the power to disrupt your life, at the present time and probably into the future. The illness not only attacks you when you are weakest but it allows other illnesses to attack at the same time. How does one fight an enemy such as this?

Summary of Illness Strengths

- Most powerful when attacks in large numbers, multiple infectious organisms damage large amounts of organ tissue.
- Able to adapt to new medications by changes in its own structure or function.
- Can sometimes be insidious, symptoms are not present until after it becomes more powerful.
- Enters and causes damage through a variety of sites, respiratory, gastrointestinal, skin, or urinary tract.
- Damage is cumulative, builds up over time, for example, high cholesterol or diabetes.
- Gains strength through hospital infections and medical errors.

Enemy Weaknesses

We need to realize that even the strongest enemy has weaknesses. How we recognize these weaknesses and use them to our advantage rests on a well-documented battle plan. In most instances, the illness is recognized and named through the use of multiple diagnostic technologies. Recognizing and naming the enemy is a key first step in any battle plan. Medical science has a researched history and a record of what offensive weapons have been the most successful. There are trained professionals who have fought against the illness, learned about its strengths and weaknesses, and hopefully have a record of success against it.

Constant evaluation can ascertain if the enemy, the illness, is contained or growing in strength. This dimension of the battle is one in which you, the patient, and family members can play an important role. Assessment skills are the key to preventing the enemy from gaining strength. They can be learned by everyone. A basic concept of this book is the teaching of these crucial assessment skills. If you add your observations and knowledge to the expertise of the professional, you have a very powerful team to fight the battle against illness. Yes, your illness is a formidable foe, but as any good soldier knows, every foe has weaknesses and battle plans key in on those weaknesses.

Summary of Illness Weaknesses

- Research has provided a record of how the illness behaves - its causes, transmission, and treatments.
- Most vulnerable when caught early when it can be treated.
- Susceptible to ongoing advances in therapies.
- Early assessment of possible complications keeps the illness visible and not hidden where it does the most damage.
- Elimination of hospital infections and medical errors prevents the illness gaining in strength.

SECURING ALLIES

You need allies! You cannot do it alone. Just as you are clear about who the enemy is, you need to identify, understand and maximize the use of your allies. A list is a wise beginning:

- Family
- Friends
- Advocates
- Nurses
- Doctors
- Religious Leaders

- Community Groups
- Media
- Fellow Hospital Families
- Insurance Company
  (Dual role: ally and
  potential adversary)

However, just naming allies is not sufficient, they need to be a part of your battle plan and their strengths and weaknesses need to be recognized. We'll start with the individuals that you choose. Who in your network of family and friends will be most supportive and helpful? Basically, who do you like having around? Whom do you trust? You are looking at the deployment of your troops.

Family

You probably will start with your spouse or best friend. Will they be able to be with you for long periods of time? One person has only so much available time and resources. Therefore, it will be better to have a team that can map out both hospital time and on-call time. It is very comforting to know you're not alone. Will these individuals be active advocates, involved in your care or quiet, silent companions, alert to change and complications? Some of us prefer privacy and have a desire to be alone, but we are talking about safety, and your plan needs to be able to reconcile your individual preferences with your survival. So, think carefully about those troops.

Coverage Schedule

Plan round-the-clock coverage for the first 24 to 48 hours if the hospital stay involves surgery or complex treatments and medications. Get a few night people who don't mind spending the late shift in a chair to monitor the patient's post-surgical state. This is particularly crucial if you have any doubts concerning the registered nurse to patient ratio. Sleep in the ICU/CCU waiting room and use your designated time with your family member to also talk with the staff. Check with the hospital policy on overnight stays and insist on your right to stay! Stay out of the way of the caregivers. You're not there to interfere with care or to be a critic but to serve as an adjunct to quality care.

Limit social visitors if they interfere with patient healing, but have a designated visitor for all shifts. If you feel comfortable with the quality of the nursing care both day and night, the extended coverage may not be necessary, but remember that deaths do occur at night during the shortest staffing periods. Questions to ask the staff:

- How often will my husband or wife be checked at night?
- Will vital signs be checked every two hours?
- Is a registered nurse on the night shift?
- How many patients is she responsible for?
- Are interns and residents on call for the night shift?

Advocate

This is a very important piece of your battle plan. You may want to choose an assertive or aggressive friend to speak for you but this type of personality may alienate the potential allies you need in order to win the battle against your illness. Assertiveness is important but it often engenders anger or defensiveness. What is the best way to be assertive in a situation where you are vulnerable? These strategies need to be clear for you, your family and your advocate. Discuss this book with your team and advocates.

Every expert advises choosing an advocate. Good plan, but why not choose several advocates: one to help you get information before the hospital admission, several to be with you during crucial phases of your hospitalization, and a business advocate to be the lead person in sorting out billing and insurance. As we emphasized before, a team best utilizes the strengths of all its members. In your planning phase you also need to designate a health care proxy with your wishes and understand the legal ramifications of both this proxy and living wills. You need to be prepared for any eventuality and make your wishes known.

How to Ask Questions

Let's look at a hypothetical situation. Someone comes to your house as a guest. You don't know the person very well but not long after the introductions, they begin to criticize your décor, how you raise your children, and your ability as a homemaker.

- *I'm really amazed that you chose peach as your living room color. I found in Better Homes and Gardens that this should always be a secondary color.*

- *It's so different to see children running around the house, out of control, but I'm sure you have your reasons.*

- *Clutter doesn't seem to bother you.*

How do you feel? What right do they have to criticize you? You're the expert on your home and family. Take this scenario to an office. A client begins by complaining about your answering service; then horror of horrors, your credentials.

- *I do hope you understand insurance law, since I see you just graduated from a small, local law school.*

- *Most lawyers seem to settle near the court house. I was surprised to find you way out here in a shopping center.*

The human response is to become defensive and justify your choices. What right do they have to criticize me? Health care workers are human. Of course, you say! But let's use that insight to develop strategies for you and your team that don't alienate the caregiver. Remember you want them to be your allies, since you are in a dependent position. Assertiveness is a valuable skill, but it needs to be used in appropriate situations.

Helpful Messages

"I messages" are much more effective since they hook in the caregiver for all the reasons they choose their profession. Critics don't get allies. Which of the following statements do you think will get the response you need?

1. *You nurses never answer my call light. I can't believe the hospital lets you get away with this sloppy care.*

2. I really feel very anxious in the hospital, and I may be pushing the call light too often, but could you help me know what's the best way to get help?

I'd pick number 2. You have given an "I message" of need, asked for help, highlighted your concern, and brought a problem into discussion.

We're not talking about crisis or emergencies, or completely inadequate care. We'll discuss strategies for those situations under the topic entitled *Chain of Command*. You and your advocate, if you use one, need to be clear on how to get the best care.

Professional Allies

Nurses and doctors are the two allies that you need to incorporate into your battle plan. Not only do you need to know their roles, but you also need to know the personality variables that make them unique. Just as you need to know your own strengths and weaknesses and those of the enemy, you need to know the strengths and weaknesses of your allies. Generalities can serve to give us a broad sense of personality variables and a better understanding. There are always exceptions to rules. You may note that your doctor or nurse is different, but this is a composite picture obtained through years in the health care system. The authors have observed and interacted with the professionals whom you need to secure as your allies.

Registered Nurses

RN's are the heart and soul of any hospital. Too dramatic and an overstatement of reality? Not really, if you have ever been hospitalized. They are your key allies, they are with you 24/7 and any successful battle plan utilizes knowledge of the major allies' strengths and weaknesses. For the purposes of this book, we will use the feminine pronoun to designate nurses. This, again, is done to eliminate the awkward she/he pronoun, but with up-front acknowledgment of the key roles male nurses hold in the profession. Traditionally, the largest numbers of nurses are female, but the definition of the word *nurse* is not gender-specific.

When you are hospitalized, you need to know the name of the registered nurse who is responsible for your care. She may not be doing your bedside care, but the quality of her supervision and case management is directly related to the success of your battle plan.

Not to mix my metaphors, but it's often very difficult to tell the players in the health care system without a scorecard. There are licensed practical nurses, aides, and technicians who can be trained to give excellent bedside care. However, the registered nurse is educated through a baccalaureate, associate degree or diploma program. This enables her to not only provide skilled bedside care, but she has the ability to coordinate the complexities of your care. She has taken the state board examination and is registered in her state to give nursing care. Your first line of defense in your battle plan is to find out the name of the registered nurse and meet with her as your chief ally. Ask questions and consult with her as she makes the rounds of her patients in the morning and checks on you before she leaves her shift. Don't hesitate to ask to talk to her if you have any concerns about your care. And, above all, treat her with respect. She is not your servant or your maid. She is your comrade in this battle.

The head nurse, now usually called the nurse manager, is often on the day shift. The charge nurse, assigned by the nurse manager, covers the evening or night shift. You need to know who they are, since the charge nurse usually changes from shift to shift. Charge nurses are trained to make assessment rounds on all the patients on the unit after receiving report. She checks the status of the patient, both physical and psychological. It is a brief contact, but is reassuring to know she is cognizant of everything going on in her unit as the nurse manager in charge.

The registered nurse assigned to your care may delegate your actual physical care but should supervise and assess the quality of your care.

Clinical instructors traveling from unit to unit in a hospital can tell very quickly the status of care and functioning of the unit by observing the charge nurse and her relationship with the RNs and staff members. You recognize the leader who is always aware of the condition of every patient on her unit and works with her team to maximize quality care.

Nursing Shortage

One serious problem that is really inherent in the system is that there is a shortage of registered nurses. This is not news, but is of great concern. We listed the warning headlines in newspapers about errors and deaths. Interestingly, at the same time, the following headlines were in the Albany *Times Union* and signal a serious dimension of the problem:

"Study Warns Shortage of Nurses Will Persist"
"Stress Will Add to Nurse Shortage, Survey Says"
"Nursing Shortage Grows"
"Nation's Care Givers Feel Crunch"
"Nurses: Increases in Staffing Levels Advised"
"The Nursing Squeeze"

Two research studies, reported in the New England Journal of Medicine in 2002 and 2003 focus on the key role of registered nurses. In May 2002, researchers concluded that a higher proportion of hours of nursing care provided by RN's and a greater number of hours of care by RN's per day was associated with better care for hospitalized patients. The 2003 study found that patients benefit most from RN care. Medical patients with the greatest proportion of RN care, relative to LPN and aides, were 9% less likely to suffer shock or cardiac arrest and develop pneumonia.

Clinical Instructors

Clinical instructors in nursing often commented that we were teaching quality care to the nurses who would care for us as we got old and gray. However, sufficient registered nurses are not there now, and it is predicted that there will be even less of these key allies when we need them the most. I don't know about you, but that is of grave concern and one of the reasons why you need to assume a portion of the nurse's role, particularly in assessment and monitoring in order to have a successful hospitalization.

As a clinical instructor, I was a second pair of eyes and provided clinical expertise as I supervised the procedures and medication administration of the student. I also made it a key point in learning to involve the patient in a three-way dialogue about what was being done. It forced the student to cognitively verbalize what she was doing and why and it was a powerful message to the patient that he or she was a partner in the care and could ask any questions. I can't be with the reader as a clinical instructor, but through the questions and examples in this book, I hope to coach you in strategies to make your voice heard. Look to me as your field manual instructor.

Not only does the nursing shortage put you at risk but it is extremely frustrating to the nurses who are stretched thin and cannot give you the kind of care that they were trained to give. Many nurses leave the bedside because they are "burned out". This may appear not to be your problem, but it is. A major premise of this book is that you are knowledgeable about your own treatments, therefore you can be the eyes of the nurse in assessment. It protects you, and the data you give the nurse will help her do her job; a partner in care is an asset. A critic of care is a liability. Nurses who are treated with respect by patients, doctors and the hospital stay in nursing.

Nurses really want to help - the profession is based on caring for those in need. When you recognize your own vulnerability and verbalize it, you will tap into the nurse's need to help. Asking to share in your care, as preparation for discharge, will build on the nurse's basic training as a health care educator. Criticizing will alienate your chief ally. Viewing your care as a collaborative relationship will maximize your success in this war. If you still have concerns about your care after your ongoing dialogue with your nurse, you have a right to discuss this with the nurse manager and go up the chain of command.

Doctors

For the purposes of this book, we will refer to doctors in the masculine pronoun. It is a simpler literary approach and eliminates the awkward he/she pronoun. Over half of the physicians in this country are now female, but many of the masculine power dimensions still reside in the title *doctor*. The training and expectations of both genders in medicine are the same in our society.

For years, doctors had a somewhat "God-like" persona. You never questioned them and were grateful that they would take care of you. As society changed, this God-like aura eroded very quickly and the respect the profession has enjoyed has lessened considerably. We don't expect God, but rather an expert physician who inspires confidence in his choice of therapies. The question for the doctor is how he can convey expertise, knowledge and competence with approachability. At the same time, no one really wants to be God anymore; it is too much responsibility, but professionals need respect for expertise. The key to working with doctors is to question them respectfully. You want answers and there are ways to get them.

Proper bedside manner! What is that? Every patient wants it and medical schools are now incorporating it in their curriculum. They have found that a good doctor/patient relationship leads to a smaller number of lawsuits. Doctors genuinely want to help patients but their ability to interact in a caring manner is almost entirely based on any

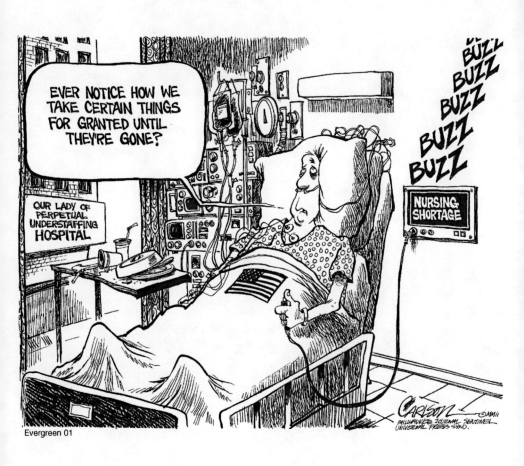

Evergreen 01

29

natural empathetic ability they have. Some do it wonderfully well, while others don't even try. The questions you need to ask are:

- *What do I need from my doctor? If he doesn't seem to be very caring, does he treat me with respect? If he expects respect from me, it should be reciprocal. I will not tolerate rudeness or being patronized.*

- *Should the criteria I use to judge my doctor be his clinical skills or his personality? No one wants a doctor who sympathetically holds your hand as you die instead of using his expertise to save you.*

- *If the doctor doesn't meet my genuine caring, supportive needs, where do I go to get these met?*

Many doctors today are burned out and feel unappreciated. One doctor told us recently how pleasantly surprised he was when a patient called to say how much she appreciated the care she had received. This section is not a plea to feel sorry for doctors, they are well compensated. Rather, it is a framework to understand motivation and allow you to use this understanding to your best advantage. It's not our job as patients to boost up their egos, but fostering a genuine relationship with allies helps you win the war.

What about doctors' egos? It takes a great deal of ego strength, dedication and perseverance to complete more than ten years of medical school, internship and residency. They are literally taught to know everything in their field and they will be penalized for not knowing. This leads to a type of personality that views questions as a threat to their expertise. How do you as a patient ask the questions that you need to have answered without triggering that defensive, threatened response, "Who are you to question me?" It can be done. Ask the questions positively but also emphasizing their responsibility to make sure you understand what is planned and any possible complications. That is informed consent, and many a malpractice suit has resulted from incomplete communication and doctors now realize this.

- *I know, Doctor, that you want me to understand the planned surgery, treatment, procedure, test, but I'm still unclear about my recovery time.*

- *I'm not questioning your expertise, Doctor, but I am having trouble understanding this complex procedure.*

- *I just need some time to discuss this with my family so we're all clear about what needs to be done.*

There is another fact about doctors. They feel particularly under pressure from insurance companies. Cash flow is an issue and they have to see a certain number of patients to survive. That makes time a crucial variable. If you as a patient know that time is often driving your doctor, how can you best prepare to use that time most effectively? A list of ten questions is not going to do it. But two well thought-out questions with follow up questions can get you the information you need. Doctors are human beings and the more you know about the personality of this major ally, the better. They are individuals but they all share the same educational and social pressures. You can use this knowledge to your advantage.

Doctors' Characteristics

- *Genuine desire to help patients*
- *Strong ego – needed to survive medical training*

- *Feels badgered and harassed by insurance companies*
- *Doesn't like to be questioned about medical choices*
- *Believes time is money and business demands appropriate cash flow*
- *Doesn't feel appreciated or valued by society*

Remember, if you understand medical education and the present daily pressures, you can devise a plan to maximize a successful interaction with your MD. Now the question is how can I use these characteristics to win my battle against illness, the true bottom line? Tap in the caring dimension of the physician with vulnerability statements. Don't use the malpractice word as a threat because you will not secure an ally. Use such statements as:

- *I'm having trouble understanding this concept because I'm so anxious. Would you explain it to me again?*

- *I know that your time is important to you, doctor, so I have two questions written down with two follow-up questions.*

If you recognize system and time constraints and have respect for the caregiver you can do much to secure an essential ally. We already discussed your principle allies in the fight against illness, the registered nurse, and the MD. But you also need to broaden your ally base for various stages of the battle. There are three major pools of potential allies that are not always utilized sufficiently in any battle plan:
- Community groups
- Media
- Fellow hospital families

Groups

Most books on hospital survival recommend that you do your homework before choosing a hospital. Choice is not always an option for every family, but pre-hospitalization research gives you an edge by letting your only hospital know you are an educated consumer and are putting them on notice that you expect high standards of care. The homework suggested by most authors is intimidating:

- *Who do I call?*
- *What questions do I ask?*
- *What is the meaning of all the data I receive?*

It can often be frustrating and not geared to meet your needs.

A better approach is to enlist the existing group that you presently belong to in a concentrated, planned evaluation of the hospital system. It could be a social group, bowling, bridge, sports, a church group, a Senior Citizens group - the possibilities are endless. It's a fact, there is strength in numbers and a group maneuver is often powerful and effective. The group makes a plan, delegates contacts and designs questions to ask each agency. One way to get this information is to use the media since many television stations and newspapers have health reporters. Enlist their help as allies to obtain this information for the well being of the community. They are looking for by-lines, air and print time. Hospitals, as all organizations, want positive publicity. If it is negative, they won't like it, but we have a right to know.

When hospitalized, make contact with other family members and patients, not just for social support but for a sharing of knowledge. How many times do students in school share information about teachers or employees share insights into employer behavior in the workplace?

- *Watch out for Mrs. Jones, she gets very upset if you talk in class.*

34

- *It will really reflect on your record if you come late to work when Arthur is the manager.*

If you are in a vulnerable situation, you need to share tips and ideas with others that have to deal with the same power structure. Talk to families you meet in the hospital and in the waiting rooms and to the family of the other patient in your hospital room. It is sad to see families in an ICU waiting room, locked in their own anxiety and not able to give each other support and valuable knowledge. View these families as your allies and maximize your power as a group.

Insurance Homework

This piece of the system is often viewed as the big, bad, uncaring corporate enemy that controls your health care. The reality is that insurance is a major player in hospitalization but a confrontational view of its usefulness will lessen your ability to focus on the true enemy, your illness. As individuals, we only have so much energy, and it should be focused on getting well, not on pre-conceived views of battles yet to be fought.

If your insurance company is viewed as your ally in getting well, then you can maximize your understanding of how to get what you need. Not necessarily what you "want", but what you absolutely need to defeat your enemy, the illness.

The first step in utilization is planning. Have you read your health insurance policy? What does it cover? Are you willing to pay more for expanded coverage or does your policy provide good coverage and care within certain boundaries? Insurance policies are extremely confusing and complete with legal and insurance terminology. You need to contact the proper personnel in the company and ask for clarification of terms and coverage. Don't be satisfied with generalities and continue with questions until you are satisfied. Do this before you need to use it and ask questions every year to find out if there have been any changes. They probably will refer you back to your policy for lists of hospitals and doctors, but days of coverage, procedures and more clarification of the appeal process are often needed. No surprises after your hospital stay!

Insurance companies offer a variety of plans. Check your personal insurance for exact coverage.

The more you know the system, the better you can make the system work for you. A general review of insurance "products" can help you determine where your policy fits in. If you are self-insured or don't have medical insurance, you need to examine what your options are in society's "safety net" (whatever that is). We wish we could fight that inequity but it is beyond the scope of this book. It seems to be beyond everyone's scope.

Companies choose health insurance plans by balancing service and cost. The latter, cost, is often the deciding factor. Questions to ask before hospitalization are:

- *Are there sufficient quantity and quality of doctors and hospitals to allow me reasonable choices?*
- *How is hospital length of stay calculated in my plan?*
- *Explain the appeal process and how I can use it.*
- *Which hospitals are par (covered) by my insurance plan?*
- *What phone calls are required prior to admission?*
- *What procedures require pre-certification?*
- *Does my doctor participate in your insurance plan?*
- *How many hospital days am I allowed for conditions if there are no complications?*

- *Is all of my care covered? Are there any excep-tions*
- *Is there any deductible?*
- *What if the insurance company denies my stay, am I responsible? (to the hospital)*

Read your policy, including the fine print, well before you need to be in the hospital. When you've done your homework about insurance companies, forget about it during your hospital stay and fight the present day battle of survival. Let the doctor and hospital follow the rules for reimbursement as they give you the best possible care.

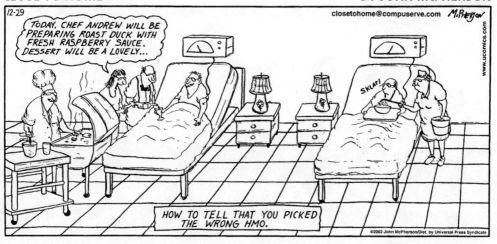

CHAIN OF COMMAND

Power Structure

In any army, there is a hierarchy and a defined chain of command with role responsibilities and status. It is clearly defined whom you report to and in turn, who reports to you. A soldier does not violate this chain of command, and if he does, there are consequences! It clarifies roles and in a battle it forms the key basis for orders to attack, retreat, deploy, engage. In the heat of battle, if your direct superior were lost, you would report to the next highest officer or non-commissioned officer. The highest-ranking officer should have the greatest experience and knowledge in order to ensure the safety of his troops.

Hospitals have similar hierarchies and knowledge of these roles is directly related to your safety. Until recently, the doctor was considered the general, with subsequent status and power. In the present health-care system, the power has clearly shifted and the CEO and CFO have clearly taken over the role of general. Physicians report to them either directly or indirectly through their chief of staff. The doctor could be considered in the role of major, a high rank, but still reporting to his superiors. This is still a prestigious and powerful position. The registered nurse would assume the role of lieutenant, first lieutenant or second lieutenant, according to training and xpertise. The nurse manager, a registered nurse, is the colonel and these officers are on the battle line with you all day, every day.

The sergeants are the licensed practical nurses and technicians that give care and possess certain technical skills. The lives of many a soldier is dependent on the savvy of their sergeants. The privates are really the backbone of any good army, and in the hospital hierarchy they would be the aides and auxiliary personnel that keep the units running smoothly. One private of special note is the ward secretary. He or she knows everything about the ward and the personnel. Their function as a communication bridge can be a valuable ally for questions of a non-medical nature. How the system functions is often dependent on the skills of the ward secretary.

You need to know all the personnel who are caring for you and their role and where they fit in the hierarchy. A nurse's aide can give you excellent bedside care, but she should not be administering medications in any form in an acute care setting. Find out who administers medications in any long-term facility that your family uses. They may allow LPN's to administer medications but you need to know how they are trained and supervised by a registered nurse. The tension in hospital care is that the hospital wants to save money by utilizing less highly trained and educated workers. These workers are trained for specific tasks by the hospital, but no matter how skilled they are, they lack the comprehensive knowledge base of the RN. If you have any doubts, check out the credentials of the caregiver in a non-critical manner. It is wise to check with the admitting RN to understand who does what on the unit. As a lieutenant, she should know. It will show that you are aware of the various roles and responsibilities.

The licenses of doctors and nurses document what they can and cannot do. A nurse cannot diagnose illness or prescribe medicine. Nurse practitioners who have intensive education in these areas can diagnose and write prescriptions, but many nurse practitioners work outside of the hospital. One other role in health care is the physician's assistant (P.A.) who has medical training and answers directly to a physician or a physician group, e.g. orthopedics, neurology. The P.A. is highly knowledgeable in that area. You will often see them making post-operative rounds and they are considered to be an adjunct to an MD. They report directly to the major (the MD) and can be considered as staff personnel rather than in a line position.

All staff must have identification badges with their name and role. If they don't ask why and find out who they are.

Territory Battles

Along with roles, comes a concept called territoriality. This is often clearly demonstrated in the MD/Nurse professional relationship. The question is how does territoriality affect you as a patient? Territoriality is the behavior pattern of an individual defending his turf (in reality, his or her scope of responsibility and status). In health care, it is manifested by protecting the exclusivity of certain skills and status, for example, "Only a nutritionist should discuss a diet with a patient." " The patient belongs to the doctor." "Only a nurse should start IVs." Scope of legitimate practice is a real concern, but when egos substitute for cooperation, the patient suffers.

Ownership

One clinical story involves a clear example of territoriality. A registered nurse was caring for a thirty six year-old man dying from pancreatic cancer. He had a wife and three small children and the nurse was supportive and looking at all aspects of potential care. She suggested to the Doctor that it would help the family if the patient was referred to hospice. The Doctor's response was, "No way, I'm not finished with him yet."

That response always angers me. The Doctor (and I hate to capitalize his name) was declaring I make these decisions, no nurse is going to tell me what to do, and I own this patient, he's mine and I decide. If I was the nurse, I would have confronted the Doctor and found another way to get the referral.

No one should own a patient, and you and your family should be alert to signs of territoriality and ownership. I don't know if they ever got to hospice, I hope they did.

Statements such as, "I know what's best for you", "It's not necessary to have a consult", "I know how to do this, I don't need to call in my nurse manager", "Interns are doctors and you need to trust me" – all should raise a red flag!

Your response to statements such as this should be:

I'm sure, Doctor, that you want what's best for me, but I need to understand what is being planned so I can give full consent to the procedure.

As reported in the April, 2004 <u>Modern Healthcare</u>, the *Institute for Safe Medication Practice*, found that intimidation by doctors prevented nurses and pharmacists from voicing concerns about the correctness or safety of medication. Physicians were more likely to use condescending language with requests from nurses rather than pharmacists. Nurses are trained to ask questions and even refuse to give medications if they have serious concerns, based on the available literature on the drug. The chain of command should encourage dialogue about safety, not discourage it with abrupt, condescending language. You, as a patient, deserve this care.

Collegial teamwork and consultations go a long way to ensure safety and you have a right to expect it. Registered nurses have to be very careful not to exceed their role responsibilities. They learn early that their professional responsibility is "don't criticize MD's". This is difficult at times, but there are channels to report any incompetence. Both doctors and nurses have an ethical professional responsibility to immediately challenge any obvious break in technique or immediate danger to a patient. Look to your nurse as your support and ask questions about all the systems that have an impact on your care. Registered nurses are highly trained and should be involved in decision-making issues. A surgeon was heard telling a nurse, "I am the authority on this." The nurse replied, "Doctor, you are the authority, but you also have a responsibility to make sure I understand what you are going to do so the patient understands."

The key to understanding the chain of command in a hospital is to know how to get immediate help. Don't do it for small matters, but if you have genuine concerns about your safety, go higher than the person at the bedside. It can be done in a non-confrontational matter.

- *I'm confused about why I'm getting this new IV. I'd like to discuss it with my doctor to better understand this treatment before we start.*

- *You've given me excellent care, but I am anxious about the procedure and Ms. Randolph, the nurse manager, said she would be available for questions.*

- *I know as an intern, you are a trained physician, but I need to talk to my attending physician to understand why this is needed.*

- *My husband's vital signs are deteriorating. I'm concerned for his life, and if a doctor does not evaluate him within ten minutes I will call our attending physician.*

If it's an emergency situation for your family member and their condition seems to be worsening, get help instantly. Stand at the nurses' station, emphasize the seriousness of your observations, and persist until a RN comes to assess the situation. Don't use this intervention because you are upset with the food or the call light is not answered immediately. Save it for the emergency. After reading this book, you'll know what warrants going beyond the chain of command. You will have the assessment skills and knowledge of your care that will enable you to recognize the signs and symptoms of serious, potentially deadly complications.

The chain of command is not always as obvious in a hospital as in the military but nevertheless it does impact both your care and safety. Use it to your advantage. These professionals should help you get an appropriate response.

Ask questions that indicate that you understand the system and are knowledgeable in your care, and can make the chain of command work for you. The key questions you need to be prepared to ask when you are hospitalized are:

- *Will a registered nurse be responsible for my care during every shift?*

- *Who is the head nurse or charge nurse on this unit during each shift - days, evenings and nights?*

- *Do you have a nursing supervisor who oversees all patient units on every shift?*

- *How are the interns and residents supervised during evening and night shifts?*

- *Will you be able to get a medical doctor to respond quickly if my husband experiences any complications?*

CHOOSING A BATTLE SITE

Physician Input

Ask your doctor when choosing a hospital. Even if the doctor does give you an answer, you also need to go to other sources. Patients often believe that they have to go to a particular hospital because their doctor wants them to go there. Remember that doctors often have privileges at several local hospitals and you need to know why he recommends that particular one. Let's hope it is not because he could not get privileges at more than one hospital or, worse yet, has lost his privileges. You certainly do not want to hear that it is nearer to his home. The argument that it has interns and residents may, in reality, be an asset for the physician who does not want to come in as often or in emergencies. Is it an asset to you and your patient care?

Surgeons logically prefer hospitals in which they are familiar with the operating room, including equipment and personnel. Familiarity and comfort can be important concerns, but you need to know the quality of post-operative care, staffing ratios, and the hospital's history of nosocomial infections. Nosocomial infections are defined as infections acquired during hospitalization or stays in a health care facility. The question is how does one get trustworthy information? Where do you look next?

Magnet Hospitals Status

Magnet hospitals are those institutions that have been given this status, after a rigorous, multifaceted evaluation by the American Nurses Credentialing Center (ANCC) (www.ancc@ana.org). It is considered the "gold standard" of nursing excellence and at the present time, only two percent of hospitals nationally, 143 hospitals out of 6,000, have achieved it. There are 95 criteria that the hospital must meet in areas including staff education, decision making, and number/type of errors. Research has shown that magnet hospitals consistently deliver better patient outcomes, spend more time at the bedside of patients, have lower death rates, and higher patient satisfaction.

If you can, have magnet status high on your list of criteria for hospital selection. Ask your hospital if they intend to seek it and when. Pressure from the consumer should demand excellence. Check the American Nurses Association Web site www.ANA.org.

Quality Assurance Department

Contact the quality assurance departments at your local hospitals. The specific information that you want should include: staffing ratios, the number of registered nurses to patients on all wards and, in particular the unit to which you will be admitted, for example, orthopedic surgery or coronary care. If you are being admitted for coronary bypass surgery, you want to know the staffing ratio in both the Intensive Care Unit and the Coronary Care Unit because you could be in either or both. Recommendations concerning appropriate nurse/patient ratios are constantly being evaluated. They are directly related to intensity of care. Some general figures for your personal battle plan:

ICU/CCU – One nurse to one to two patients
Pediatrics – One nurse to four patients
Medical/Surgical – One nurse to six patients

Check with the American Nurses Association and your state nurses association for their recommendations.

This is also the time to ask about the infection rate in the operating room and on the units as this is the key question and you need specific answers. A hospital quality assurance department has data but unless required by law, they do not share it. Ask the questions anyway to put pressure on hospitals to disclose. Just the thought of obtaining this level of information can be very intimidating and overwhelming. The tendency is to just trust one's luck and hope for the best. But this type of thinking does not contribute to your battle plan and help you to win the war.

What you need to do is enlist the help of those groups and media allies that we discussed previously. Groups are powerful and the responsibility for this daunting task of obtaining information should be shared. Tasks and questions should be delegated and a method of reporting back to all the members established. You have enlisted a group in your battle plan and the following questions will help you rate hospitals.

This is where you and your group use your best assertive behavior. If they bombard you with facts and figures, ask them for the specific data, how does their hospital compare to state and national norms on standards of care, infection rates and medical errors?

Hospitals may resent these types of questions, but a good hospital will have this information available, since state regulators and accreditation agencies for hospitals require it. This can't be emphasized enough. If more consumers, patients and families requested information, it would generate more accountability. Many states and the federal government, through Medicare, are now requiring infection rate information be made public.

Sample Battle Plan for Choosing a Hospital Site

❑ The hospital's quality assurance or risk management department. Ask specific questions and be persistent, note how they reply:

- *Number of reported infections on units.*

- *Infection rate for operating room.*

- *Have you ever had units closed because of infections, when did this happen and what did you do about it?*

- *How many reportable medical errors have you had?*

- *What is your hospital protocol for ongoing training in error prevention?*

- *How does your hospital compare to the state and national norms for reportable errors?*

- *Who controls the number of hours that your interns and residents work? How many continuous hours do they work?*

In 2004, two <u>New England Journal of Medicine</u> articles reported on student doctors and medical errors. Those who worked no more than 16 hours without a break made about one third fewer serious errors. Overworked interns, working more than 80 hours a week, made 21 percent more serious medication errors and 34 percent more serious errors overall than colleagues who worked fewer hours. They may be excellent doctors, but they need less hours of work and more supervision. Factor this in when you choose a hospital.

❑ State health department:

- *What are the state requirements and criteria for reporting hospital infections and errors?*

- *Do you have a rating of hospital on both nosocomial infections and medical errors.*

- *What are the state regulations for registered nurse / patient ratios?*

❑ Joint Commission on Accreditation of Healthcare Organizations (JCAHO). Website: www.JCRINC.com

- *What area hospitals are accredited?*

- *If any hospital was on probation or not accredited, what was the reason, when did it occur and what did they do to get accredited?*

- *What data do you have on hospital infections and medical errors in specified hospitals?*

❑ American Nurses Association, Phone: 1-800-274-4ANA, Website: www.ANA.org

- *What are your recommendations for registered nurse/patient ratios?*

- *What are your recommendations on forced overtime?*

- *Do you provide nurses with guidelines for preventing infection and preventing nursing errors?*

☐ American Medical Association (AMA), Phone: 1-800-262-3211, Website: www.AMA-ASSN.org

- *What are your recommendations for supervision of interns and residents?*

- *Does the association recommend the number of hours interns and residents should work?*

- *What guidelines have you prepared to help physicians prevent nosocomial infections and medical errors?*

☐ Medicare, Phone: 1-800-252-6550, Website: www.Medicare.gov

Internet

Use the Internet to obtain background information, but remember what is put on the web will be positive data. The web can be an invaluable asset, however, be sure to check the credentials of any site on the Internet. Remember hospital web sites are in reality advertisements for each hospital's strong points. They will not list the units that have been closed because of infection. Your state health department, the accrediting organization for hospital review, and private health care sites have more objective data.

☐ The website www.hospitalcompare.hhs.gov provides side by side hospital vs. hospital comparisons on 17 measures related to heart attack, heart failure and pneumonia care. The same information can be obtained from 1-800-Medicare.

This hospital comparison website was just unveiled and will be updated quarterly, 4,200 hospitals are listed.

❑ The Agency for Healthcare Research & Quality (AHRQ) has awarded their Distinguished Hospital Award to 135 U.S. hospitals based on patient safety (www.healthgrades.com). This site does not list information on hospitals that have poor records. Community research by local groups is still crucial to get information that will be most helpful to you and apply pressure for quality care.

Type of Hospital

One dimension of the decision concerning a hospital often involves the choice between a community hospital, medical center, or hospital with a national reputation. Each one has advantages and also disadvantages.

Community hospitals have a more familiar presence, are smaller, with local reputations. Often it is the hospital your family has used for generations. It might be run by a particular religion, and there is the comfort of familiarity. They often have a more stable staff that does not have as high a turnover rate as in a medical center. That can be an advantage. One disadvantage would be if the facility does not have the specialists or technology to care for your particular illness.

Medical centers have a wide variety of specialists and cutting-edge technology. This may be what you absolutely need. They are often teaching hospitals and the staff will be knowledgeable in the newest techniques and therapies. The disadvantages include your lack of familiarity with the facility and the basic intimidation factor of a large medical center. There is also a greater turnover of staff in a medical center. You will have to ask yourself if you are comfortable being cared for by interns and residents. They can be the most skillful and caring physicians. Remember these questions:

- *Will in-house staff care for me?*
- *How are they supervised?*
- *How many hours do they work?*

You don't want tired, inexperienced interns and residents.

Nationally recognized health centers pose some unique challenges. It is clear they are experts in their field and have done multiple surgeries and protocols in your illness area. One essential criterion in choosing a surgeon is how often he or she has done the procedure. You can assume that the nationally known hospital is experienced in the surgery, but you cannot assume that the facility gives high-level care and has a low rate of hospital-based infections.

Your choice of a battle site is done carefully, but sometimes you find you need or prefer going to a nationally acclaimed medical center. You want to be with the best, or so you think. If your local hospital is confusing and intimidating, the large, prestigious medical center is overwhelming. You are less familiar with the players, the chain of command and back-up system. If you are admitted to a hospital outside of your geographic area, your understanding of your resources is more complex but absolutely critical.

In 2002, a 57 year-old newspaper reporter died at a nationally known transplant center, three days after donating part of his liver to his critically ill brother. As reported in the Albany *Times Union*, the N.Y.S. Health Commissioner called the post-operative care sloppy; there was a lack of adequate nursing and medical staffing, lack of communication among staff, failure to identify abnormal symptoms, and failure to respond immediately when the patient's condition continued to deteriorate.

What was particularly chilling about this report was how desperately the family had tried to get help when they knew their loved one was not doing well. The newspaper report stated the many times the wife tried to get help for her husband but the system failed them. The intimidation factor of a nationally renowned hospital increases proportionately with its reputation. Yet, for some conditions, the only hospital that can provide the most up-to-date treatments is the large, prestigious medical center. Who am I to question the care at this prestigious center? But if I don't, who will? All the battle strategies that you implemented in your local hospital need to be used here.

You and your family are out of your support system. It is truly a "foreign battle zone". Who can you turn to for help? When you make such a decision you must have a fail-safe plan. Who do I get in touch with if the staff does not respond to my questions? Have a list of back-up telephone numbers if the chain of command is not working. On that list include the phone number of the chief resident and the attending physician. Your State health department may have an emergency number. One key back up is the right to call the referring physician in one's home area. Doctors know how to get other doctors to respond. They know the standard of care for your illness and they can agitate the system to secure a response. Use this plan in an emergency situation. There are times when we need to demand immediate attention and action. You may be considered a troublemaker, but you will get results and in this instance time is crucial.

Many individuals don't have a choice in a hospital; for example, you live in a small community or rural area. Asking questions of the hospital is still valuable. It lets them know that you are knowledgeable and that you will be vigilant and will not accept sub-par care. Quality care demands that the consumer puts pressure on the provider to have safe nurse/patient ratios and infection control plans in place.

Financing the Hospitalization

You've read your health insurance policy and one major restriction is you can't use an "out of network" hospital in your health care plan. Is the hospital "par", participating?

What hospitals does your insurance cover and what if you want the freedom to go to a different doctor and hospital? You need a policy that allows you to go out of network. If you had data that found a particular hospital unsafe because of infections, present it to the insurance company. They may deny your request; however, quality assurance is a bottom line in business. Infection causes re-admission, re-admission cost money. That hospital can be reexamined by the insurance company for compliance and accountability. You need to do your homework. Personal preference or vague tales of incompetence do not work in the insurance world. If enough consumer voices are heard demanding quality care, change can occur. You need to be armed with knowledge and data. How you deal with the insurance company if they will not pay will be examined in depth in a later section.

This is also the time to ask the hospital how they calculate costs:

I don't want to be responsible for horrendous hospital bills after discharge:

- *What does the charge for a hospital day cover?*

- *Can I assume that all nursing care, including assessment, monitoring, treatments, and the administration of medication is included in the daily rate?*

- *Are there separate calculations for drugs, laboratory work, and x-rays?*

- *What is the usual operating room cost for a total hip replacement?*

- *How does the hospital bill for anesthesia?*

- *Does my insurance cover all these charges? If not, how much do they usually cover? How many hospital days are covered for this operation?*

- *Are there any other charges that I need to calculate in my planning?*

It always amazes me that intelligent consumers who question each hotel, cable, Internet, and telephone bill do not use the same skills in planning for a hospitalization. If more health care consumers did this, there would be more hospital accountability and less "sticker shock" at discharge. Even such a perceptive analyst as Andy Rooney shared in a recent column his surprise at the cost of an overnight hospital stay. There was a State of New York surcharge of $207.98. I live in New York and never realized the state taxed hospitals the same as hotels. Isn't hospitalization as necessary as food? Most interesting, was *Miscellaneous Services*, $4,856.95. What are they, how are they calculated, and why does the insurance company pay only half of it? Does the insurance company know something we don't know? Are all the charges justified? Planning should include the collection of this type of data, to be used, if necessary, in post-discharge skirmishes.

Location

You may think that nearness to accommodations will not be of concern in a hospitalization, but consider your support network. Their job of monitoring and assessing the family member's hospitalization will be enhanced if family and friends can be a part of the team approach. Are there accommodations and restaurants they can use if distance and travel from home is a concern? A two-hour commute and fatigue will detract from their hospital presence.

Recommendations

As far as family and friends' recommendations, one should listen closely to negative concerns. A positive view of a hospital should not substitute for your homework. Aunt Mary might have had wonderful care when she was hospitalized for congestive heart failure, but you are having prostate surgery. Incidents of surgical infections are the data that are crucial to your choice. If your child is hospitalized, you need to know the specific details concerning the pediatric unit, and also their policy for allowing you to stay with the child, even to the point of the administration of anesthesia in the operating room.

Timing of Battle

Some experts recommend you time your hospitalization so you don't experience it during July, when new interns and residents begin. We take exception to this advice to avoid "elective surgery" during July and August. What is elective surgery? Should I tell my damaged hip to wait two months for repair? Should I ignore my doctor's recommendation that I have my gall bladder removed as soon as possible? Can I ignore the fact that in my company the best time to have sick time is during the summer? And we know emergencies can't wait! Instead of fixing the problem, they throw the responsibility back on the patient and family.

Our recommendation is to radically change the supervision of new interns and residents. Is it too much to ask for attending physicians to assume a more prominent role in this transition period? Realistically, you can't always pick the time of your hospitalization and statistics show that medical errors occur at all times of the year. A better approach would be to bring out in the open your concerns about personnel. Make sure your MD countersigns any decision. Let the intern and resident know that you are aware that he is new. You are supportive of learning, but you need to know who is supervising him and their communication with each other. A learning environment can be safe if the learner is supervised and there are double check procedures in place. Clinical instruction in nursing requires that the student and the clinical instructor care for the patient. The challenge in medicine is to ascertain how the interns and residents are being supervised.

If a doctor who you do not know comes to do a procedure, you need to ask the following questions: not critically, but because you are anxious and vulnerable. Begin with an "I message":

I get very anxious in the hospital and it's important for me to know who is caring for me, and their qualifications.

Continue with any or all of the following questions:

- *Are you the intern or resident on this service?*
- *Is this a procedure ordered by my attending physician?*
- *I would prefer you speak to my doctor before you do this new procedure.*
- *How long have you been on this service?*
- *How many hours have you been on call?*
- *How many times have you done this procedure?*
- *Who is your direct supervisor for orders and procedures?*

You do not have to be a guinea pig for the learner. Expect some defensiveness from the physician because as a novice they may be threatened by questions, but your questions are legitimate and the way he responds will let you know how safe you are. The most reassuring response from a doctor or nurse will be honesty. "This is a new procedure for me and if you are anxious about it let me get my supervisor (nurse manager or resident, depending on the caregiver) and he or she will supervise me." You always have the right to request a new caregiver if their response is evasive or angry. No one can know everything, and the nurse or doctor who says that they do is potentially very dangerous. **A skilled practitioner is confident in their knowledge, not threatened by questions, and always willing to consult and be open to new ideas.** They recognize that your care and comfort are the primary issue.

Any soldier knows that the site of the battle is one key to success or failure. Is it a mountain or desert terrain? Can you control the high ground? How will the climate impact your battle plan? Your pre-planning and choosing of a hospital has the same significance. Remember to include your vacation areas and those locations that you frequently visit. Illness often stages a sneak attack and you need to be ready for all contingencies.

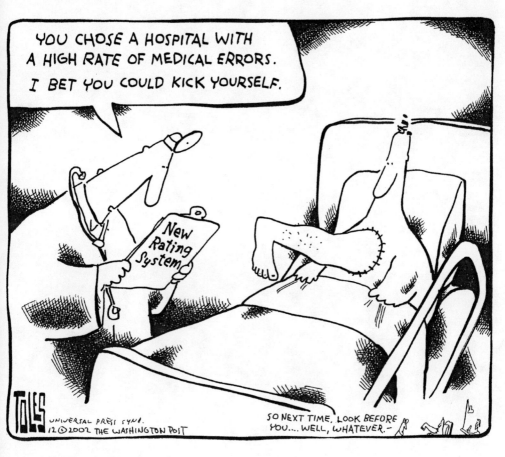

PREPARATION FOR BATTLE
FIELD MANUAL NOTES

Personal Notes:
- *Allies' and Advocates' roles, telephone numbers*
- *Questions to ask when and to whom, follow-up questions*
- *Timeline for obtaining data*
- *Names and roles of personnel, nurse manager, registered nurses, interns and residents.*
- *Chain of command, who supervises who*
- *Telephone numbers of doctors, hospital business office, Medicare, insurance company*

_____

_____

_____

_____

_____

_____

_____

_____

_____

_____

_____

PART TWO

DEPLOYMENT

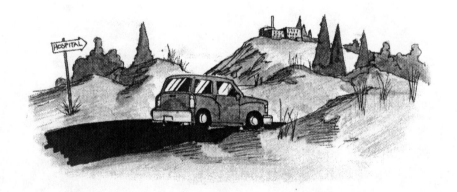

Voices:
Counselor and Teacher

STRATEGIC FIELD MANUAL

Every soldier has a field manual that includes the general principles of battle:

Soldier	Patient
• Who is your enemy	Illness
• How to secure allies	Planning Phase
• When to engage	Timing, Emergency Room
• When and how to attack or retreat	Questions, Assessment, Monitoring Skills
• What weapons will you use	Insider knowledge, Basic Skills assessment
• Number of troops needed	List of Allies

Like a soldier, when you are hospitalized, keep your field manual with you. It is intended to be the kind of book that's dog-eared from use, with coffee and juice stains and filled with notes, questions and ideas. Use it now, use it when you need it, use it over and over again. The manual provides you with strategies to keep you alive. Soldiers need to learn specific skills; techniques and maneuvers designed to help them survive - so do you. In the hospital, knowledge is power for the patient. However, too many general facts and instructions can be over-whelming and force the learner to give up. The *Engagement* section defines specific procedures that you will need to understand in order to better assess the quality of your care. Before that, we need to examine powerful weapons that you can use.

Weapons

Your greatest weapon in your battle against illness is yourself and your family. The planning you do, your knowledge of the system and quality care, and your strategic use of allies. There are also specific weapons and knowledge that you can use and we include them in your field manual as you deploy to the hospital battlefield. Understanding the language of war and the psychological dimensions of your care adds to your power.

Weapon One: Nursing Diagnosis

One of the major dimensions of the MD's role is diagnosis of illness. While the RN cannot diagnose the illness, she does formulate a nursing diagnosis. You, as the patient, should know what makes up your nursing diagnosis. The nursing diagnosis was developed to individualize nursing care. There was resistance in the profession at first, another task to add to the burden of the nurse. Now it is a basic concept of nursing, even though some nurses may do it in a routine manner.

The nursing diagnosis was developed to document the patient's response to the illness, a key concept. It is defined as a statement that describes the patient's actual or potential response to a health problem that the nurse is licensed and competent to treat. So the patient changes from "the cholecystectomy in Room 553" to "Mrs. Atkins" who has the following nursing diagnosis:

- Ineffective airway clearance after surgery related to incision pain.

  Mrs. Atkins cannot take a deep breath because her surgical wound hurts so much. If she doesn't breath deeply and cough to bring up mucus, she could develop a pneumonia. Make sure she has the proper pain medication so she can cough and deep breath.

- Feeding self-care deficit related to previous cerebral vascular accident.

Mrs. Atkins is in for surgery but since she suffered a stroke previously, she is not able to use her hands to feed herself. Make sure there is someone who can help her eat. Possible referral to occupational or physical therapy.

- Social isolation related to age and lack of family contacts.

Mrs. Atkins does not have regular visitors or potential caregivers at home after discharge. Contact social services to see about social supports; perhaps volunteers or possible church groups.

As you can see, Mrs. Atkins becomes a unique person with specific needs that translate into nursing care. The nursing diagnosis fits within the nursing process consisting of assessment, planning, implementation and evaluation. As a part of your training, you will learn assessment and evaluation skills. With these skills and knowledge of your nursing diagnosis, you can be a full partner in the implementation of your care. Ask the nurse to tell you what your nursing diagnoses are and review how they impact your care.

Weapon Two: Redundancy

In your basic training manual one needs to look at and develop a repertoire of "what if" questions. In planning and building large construction projects, engineers and architects build in safety and contingency plans. This same meticulous, additional planning should be in health care. This is called redundancy. Redundancy is defined as an overabundance, more than enough, excess, or superfluous. In designing any large project, engineers base their calculations on the highest level of strength and flexibility. Then they add in additional systems above and beyond the baseline to prepare for extra contingencies, for example, typhoon winds or severe earthquakes. In certain circumstances, more is needed and they design for unusual circumstances. In health care, there are constant unusual circumstances and we need to build in bedside redundancy.

In hospital care, there are very few redundancy plans at the bedside. Two examples in place in the hospital are:

1. The procedure that requires two nurses to check the type and cross match of the blood transfusion with the patient's information before administration and;

2. Two nurses, scrub and circulating, count the sponges in the O.R. before the incision is closed. Double checks can be done with medication calculations if the nurse requests it.

What we are proposing in this field manual is systematic redundancy using the patient and family members as the additional check for quality care. To do this potentially life-saving action, you must understand what is being done so you can question appropriately. While we are not designing a major building or bridge, we are designing a bedside plan that can save you or your family member's lives. A system of bedside "double checks" needs to be in place in the hospital setting. The staff doesn't do it for so called "routine" procedures. You need to provide this redundancy to stay alive, not get hospital infections and not be the object of medical errors.

By asking the "what if" question, the first step in setting up a plan for redundancy, you bring quality care into the foreground for discussion and emphasize accountability.

- *What if during the operation you find something unexpected, what will you do?*

- *What if the medication causes side effects, what will you prescribe?*

- *What if my IV stops running, what is the hospital procedure?*

- *What if I get a wound infection, how will it be recognized and treated?*

- *What if I have an allergic reaction to the medication, do you have emergency procedures in place?*

You may get a general response; however, ask for more specific details. The main purpose of these questions is to ascertain that the caregiver is not only aware of but also planning for all complications. One cannot predict every individual, physiological response, but you need to demand a professional who has a built in, fail-safe system and back-up plans in place.

Recently, the American College of Physicians has developed teaching models to lessen doctor errors, and one component of it focuses on cognitive failures. Cognitive refers to thinking and rational planning, recognizing that there are human cognition limits. The program proposes tools and techniques to help the physician avoid errors. The first step in examining thinking and planning is to bring the process into conscious examination. The "what if" question by the patient forces the caregiver (doctor, nurse or health care technician) to examine the routine and look at it again.

As a patient, you can't wait until all caregivers have programs on cognition and built in redundancy plans. Your life is at stake. Questions about complications and plans are valid and an appropriate tool for patient safety.

Weapon Three: Hospital Gear

As a hospital patient, you need to take "equipment" that will help you get well and fight your enemy, illness:

- Your field manual with key telephone numbers
- No valuables, there are security problems
- Personal hygiene products
- Comfortable sleep wear so you can get out of that horrible hospital gown as soon as possible
- Comfort equipment—your rosary, copy of the Bible, worry beads, a favorite book, family pictures, soft afghan, psychological security blankets
- Inexpensive earphones, tape deck and music that comforts you
- Computer, cell phone (if allowed by hospital policy); Electronic devices should be used in such a way as to not disturb your roommate.
- Antibacterial hand wipes. Offer them to visitors and health care workers. They may respond that they just washed their hands or used hospital wipes. By bringing them into your health care space, adding redundancy, you are making a statement that you are aware of hospital infections and wish to protect yourself. Hand washing, a crucial element of infection control, will be discussed in the Engagement section.

Weapon Four: Assessment Skills

You know your enemy; have lined up allies, understand the nursing diagnoses and have developed "what if" questions. Now the key skill you bring into battle is vigilant assessment. This process and skill is taught to beginning nursing students. It is knowledge that provides you with a method to keep more control of the hospitalization experience. Both you and your primary allies: family, friends and advocates, need to have this skill. You all have to be on the same page.

Assessment is the first step in the nursing process, and it is a problem-solving approach. It is the process of gathering, verifying and communicating data about a client to ascertain the level of wellness, health practices, past illnesses, and health care needs. Most textbooks state that the client is the best source of information and provides the most accurate source of health care needs. The history and physical are all part of the initial assessment but the process is constant, changing and dynamic. Every time a nurse is with a patient, she should be constantly assessing status. Since you are the source of the data, your initial reporting of signs and symptoms can alert the nurse to changes in your condition. The sooner complications are found the better the outcome, a crucial step in weakening your illness enemy.

In this time of nursing shortages, it is the wise patient and family who become their own nurses. In a care giving relationship, you are the most important participant. You will recognize crucial signs and symptoms and understand the different characteristics. Symptoms are subjective, physical sensations or psychological feelings that you are experiencing in relation to your illness. Signs are actual objective physical occurrences that can be seen. "I feel rather warm", is a symptom while ascertaining your elevated temperature is a sign. "My leg feels sore", is a symptom while redness and swelling of the leg is a sign. Both are valid statements and should be utilized in any assessment.

On some occasions, the symptoms may be somewhat vague but they need to be noted and checked. "I don't know, I feel a little shaky, I was okay this morning but now I feel uneasy." Vital signs, intake and output, condition of dressing, are all areas that need to be checked and blood work may be ordered.

The key to redundancy is that you note and describe change to the nurse. Expect the staff to act on this. For example, make sure that they monitor vital signs and temperature. As we move into the *Engagement* section of this book, all the signs, symptoms, and procedures you need to understand will be explained and highlighted.

You have planned, now it is time to learn the psychological aspects of this war, and this is crucial to your success. You can use the blank pages provided in this book to write down observations and questions for the nurse. The signs and symptoms that demand immediate action and when you need to go up the chain of command to get a life-saving response are examined in *Engagement*.

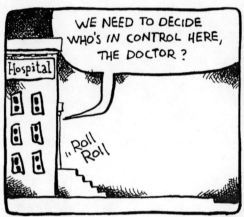
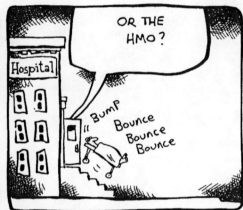
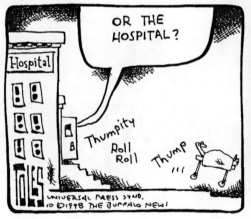
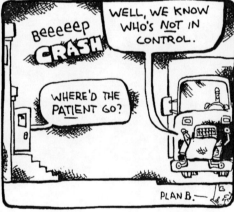

10/1/98

LANGUAGE OF WAR

You know your enemy, your allies and your hospital. The language of war surrounds you and a strategy is needed to understand and utilize it for your successful battle. I've included several clinical stories in this deployment section. I believe they illustrate important points and give you, the reader, an insight into our beliefs about caregivers and accountability. Deployment provides you with the how, why, and when of asking questions. The following sections provide you with the additional knowledge to ask further "what-if" questions.

Shorthand

One serious mistake by patients and family members is not challenging the abbreviations and jargon that health care workers use. These shortcuts in communication save time but can also lead to errors and keep you out of the loop. Every organization, profession and work place has a unique language. It gives a sense of belonging to a group and a certain status, "I know it, and you don't." In your battle for survival with a successful outcome goal, that motto is not acceptable. The health care worker may not realize they're talking in shorthand since it becomes so routine. You need to take the routine into awareness to prevent errors and help your own understanding. One can't be a member of the team if one doesn't know the language and ground rules.

It is not necessary to know what S.O.B. (short of breath), Q.I.D. (four times a day), H.S. (hour of sleep), COPD (chronic obstructive pulmonary disease), CABG (coronary artery bypass graft) means all of the time. You probably won't remember. You can't learn them all and new terms are constantly added. What you do need to know is the following sentence:

In order to get well, I need to know what you're saying, and I don't understand...please explain it to me. It's still unclear, let me write it down.

It may be a simple decoding of an abbreviation. But it can also lead you to other questions that will clarify your care. Your silence may be interpreted as understanding when, in fact, you may be too confused to ask. Don't be embarrassed to ask. Even personnel in the health care field for years can be floored by new abbreviations and jargon.

Non-Verbal Messages

Verbal language can always be questioned but you need to recognize the non-verbal messages and the labeling that can be a part of one's hospital stay. When a soldier is deployed to a foreign war zone, he is prepared with a basic understanding of the language. However, as important as that is, knowledge of the body language, gestures, tone of voice, and culture of the land will also be crucial in order to survive. A soldier needs to know the difference between friendly words and gestures, and aggressive, threatening communication, verbal or non-verbal. Language and intent are conveyed in many ways including through non-verbal messages. The purpose of this section is to bring this non-verbal and attitudinal language into the dialogue concerning your health needs. If you are not aware of the labels staff may use or of the counter-transference ambush, you are handicapped in your ability to confront it and lessen its impact on your health care. The unspoken attitudes need to be brought into the forefront.

If the caregiver becomes angry or defensive with your questions, bring this into discussion.

- *I don't understand. You seem annoyed by my questions.*

- *I know you're busy and you seem hurried and annoyed by my question. I need to understand this treatment, could you come back later when you have time?*

These questions can be used with any health care worker, doctor or nurse. Their tone of voice, posture and sighing can more accurately convey their feelings as opposed to merely answering your questions. Don't be afraid to note what you perceive, not as a criticism, but rather as an observation. They may not know what their non-verbal signs are communicating. Better to have these negative feelings discussed rather than to have the staff member go out to colleagues and label you as a complainer. Your questions are legitimate; the labeling is not.

Avoidance

Avoidance occurs when health care workers, who are unaware of their own personal feelings and bias, practice a pattern of giving the treatments and procedures that are ordered but avoiding patient contact at all other times. This avoidance is not a conscious plan but results from their all too human values. We all tend to avoid what we do not understand or view as a threat. When this occurs in health care, you are not receiving all the care, including assessment and monitoring, that is your right. I saw this very early in my professional life and it had major implications for my subsequent journey in nursing.

The Room at the End of the Hall

Picture St. Mary's Hospital, tall ceilings, wide, long corridors in both directions, and the nursing station in the middle. As a student, the setting was intimidating and every patient interaction was significant. After all these years, I can still remember one patient so vividly. She was a young woman, in her thirties, who was dying of ovarian cancer. Her room was at the end of the hall on the left, the furthest distance from the nurses' station.

In caring for her with a staff nurse, I saw that no one went into her room except when they had to give her medicine or do a treatment. She was so alone and I didn't know what to do or say. Avoidance was the norm. This was before hospice, and what we now know about caring for the dying patient. Staff avoided the dying patient because they didn't know what to say. They also identified with the young woman "What if that was me?" Too much to handle!

I know I wanted to do more but didn't know how. I decided then and there, that I was going to learn how and started my journey as a counselor. I wasn't there for her, but I wish she knew what an impact she had on my professional life. Maybe she does now.

I've included this clinical story because it was important to me and illustrates how avoidance occurs. Avoidance happens whenever a health care worker is threatened or uncomfortable with a patient for a variety of reasons: bias, lack of training or personal defense mechanisms. Whatever the cause, avoidance, this non-verbal behavior, impacts on your care and you need to recognize it and bring it into discussion. Avoidance behavior is unacceptable.

I don't understand. Everyone who cares for me seems to run in and out, no chance for questions. Is there something that I have done or said?

PSYCHOLOGICAL WARFARE

Labeling

Knowing the psychological dimensions of care gives you more ammunition, insider analysis of staff behavior that directly impacts on your survival.

When you are admitted to the hospital, you will be labeled and not always in a complimentary way. You may become any of the following:

- Good patient
- Angry patient
- Agitated patient
- Crock
- Sun downer
- Fatso
- Gomer

- MI in Room 203
- Whiner
- Complainer
- Loony
- Crazy
- Gork

Obviously, this will not be verbalized to you, but in reality it may be in the staff member's mind. It's extremely important in your hospital battle to recognize that labels exist and lessen their use with you or your family members by open discussion of needs and behavior. Bring labeling into the open.

Disruptive Patient

If your family member is particularly distraught, anxious, medically "out of it", abrasive by nature or has a mental problem, be sure to talk this over with the nurse. Even the most kind, loving individual can have personality changes in the hospital. You don't want your loved one (who, by the way, drives you crazy sometimes) to be treated less carefully because of their behavior. The label of "difficult", "crank", "crock" or worse can be applied very quickly. Better to say to the nurse,

I know my mother can be very difficult at times, but she's so upset and anxious by this hospitalization. Could we come up with some strategies to help her cope and help all of you also?

This method brings a problem into objective discussion and you can tap into professional behavior. Ignoring the behavior will impact on the quality of care your mother receives.

ICU Horror

One RN in my class described what she did with an Intensive Care Unit (ICU) patient who was "disruptive". She was very proud that she used behavior modification for one patient who screamed all the time and disturbed the other patients. When he screamed she would put a pillow over his face to stop the outburst and she reported that it worked. The pillow modified his screaming behavior.

How could any caregiver be so inhumane and also compromise the patient physiologically in a critical care unit, or any unit? The class of other nurses and myself told her, in no uncertain terms, that this was a completely inappropriate maneuver on her part, uncaring and dangerous.

The fact that she thought that she was doing something helpful was very disturbing and illustrates how health care professionals can misuse information from other disciplines. A little knowledge can be a bad thing.

This story demonstrates why families need to be proactive and question what the staff will do with certain types of disruptive behavior.

My husband seems so agitated and restless and his screams are heartbreaking to me. What are you doing to comfort him and help him to be more peaceful?

Don't assume they will take appropriate action. In many instances they will use some form of medication but there are other comfort measures that may help – back rubs, position changes, a quiet environment with less sensory stimulation.

Agitated Patient

Hospitals cause agitation in many patients, not only the elderly. The question is always, why is this happening with this individual patient? The nursing diagnosis must reflect that analysis. The following clinical story comes from our own personal experience with nursing home care.

Agnes and Irene

This story is about two elderly women who shared six years of time together in a nursing home. Irene was sweet and funny, rather cute in her own way and always called everyone "lovey". She didn't know where she was, but didn't appear to be particularly bothered by that. In fact, she informed her daughter that she was going to talk to the dean about taking some more courses.

Agnes was labeled as an "agitated" elderly patient. She could not speak, but her eyes looked trapped. She began her sojourn in the nursing home pacing the halls of her ward and when she couldn't walk anymore she pounded on the arms of her chair or tray table.

Both received good basic care, but whom do you think received extra attention and love? Irene was my mother and Agnes was my mother-in-law. It was hard to watch my mother get old and frail and lose herself but it broke my heart to watch Agnes, who could not be comforted.

Irene, the "good" patient, got extra care. The "agitated" patient, Agnes, got care, but often was ignored and received less attention, assessment, and monitoring.

Anger

It may be difficult for family members to relate to their ill-loved ones at times. Illness does strange and unpredictable psychological things to people. They're anxious, vulnerable, scared and usually very angry and this anger may or may not be expressed. We looked at constructive anger expression as a potential strength in an earlier section of this book. It needs some further discussion in deployment.

Anger at circumstances may be displaced onto the nearest available caregiver. If I can't get mad at my doctor, or this stupid illness, I can get mad at you, my husband, because you love me. Recognize that anger, appropriately expressed and used, can generate healing energy. Repressed anger, expressed inappropriately, can generate further animosity and have a negative impact on patient care.

When an individual becomes ill, they grieve for their old, healthy self as body image and self-concept changes occur. The family is angry also, at the system, illness, and even unconsciously at the family member who became ill and disrupted their lives. It isn't logical, the person did not choose to get ill, but the anger is real, normal, and a necessary part of the grieving process.

Stairway Anger

Many years ago, a dear friend's husband died of cancer. It was sudden and found during a simple hernia operation. In those days, there was no support for the family of a dying patient. There was no way for my friend to express anger, it was viewed as a negative emotion.

My friend used to leave the ICU, where she watched her husband dying, and go into the stairway of the hospital to scream and hit the walls. There was no place in the system for support, counseling and recognition of her feelings and people at that time would have thought she was crazy, probably even now. I wonder if anyone heard her.

As caregivers, we like to think we've come a long way since then in our ability to not only recognize anger, but help the patient and family express it in a healing way. I'm not so sure.

Family members need to know these feelings of anger are very normal. They need counselors, social workers and nurses who can listen to and recognize these emotions. In the long run, as family members, the sooner you understand your feelings, the better you can assume the role of a caregiver.

An angry patient can be acknowledged and helped but often they are avoided. Express your anger, not at staff, but say that you need to talk about your anger. Expressed feelings get help; unexpressed negative feelings lead to labeling and less quality care. Labeling you or your family member as an "angry" patient leads to avoidance by staff.

Using anger in a therapeutic relationship involves helping a client find ways to express anger constructively by finding an outlet and using this energy for healing. The act of writing down your feelings can serve as one outlet, and later discuss these feelings with the right person.

Some individuals, even professionals, cannot handle anger in any way, shape or form and they don't even recognize how they displace their own anger onto patients. If you sense anger toward yourself or a family member in the hospital, bring it up into discussion.

I don't understand, you seem so angry at my mother. What has she done to cause these feelings?

No patient should be subjected to an angry health care worker. It is unsafe and compromises your care.

Hospital Humor

The culture in a hospital supports a group of individuals who work together in a setting that requires multiple skills, interpersonal relating, team building and one that also can be highly stressful at any time. This can be said of multiple professions but hospitals are unique, as the staff is dealing with illness and life and death situations. There is a sense that "we're all in this together" and the outside groups or "enemy" can be administrators, doctors who come and go, families and even patients.

One staff rule is loyalty and there is a prevalent type of hospital humor that keeps staff going. Books have been written about humor and its necessity for survival but it can at times be very insensitive. Humor is a powerful life force, but humor that is at the expense of a patient and patient care is unacceptable. Viewed as a tension reliever, it has merit, but where is that insensitive line? That line occurs when the object of humor is vulnerable and lacks power in the system. My students were taught to bring instances of derogatory remarks made by staff about patients to post-conference for discussion. That was not the kind of behavior that I wanted them to model. The MASH humor on TV was against each other, the war, the system, and superiors. Hawkeye Pierce never made fun of his patients. I hope my former students always remember this. Use humor for healing.

What can a patient or family do, since jokes often occur behind closed doors, for example, at morning report? Be aware of its existence and monitor your care or family member's care. If you hear any use of it toward any family member, object immediately and strongly. True humor should not be insensitive and cruel when people are most needy and vulnerable.

Counter-Transference Ambush

You may, as the patient, experience a transference response. How many times have you felt any of the following: anxiety, confusion, guilt or anger when dealing with certain individuals? You may not know why. Often, feelings are triggered by the following people: mother, father, Aunt Helen, Sister Louise (you fill in the blanks). That's transference. Transference occurs when your positive or negative feelings toward significant others from the past are projected to the caregiver. It takes some thoughtful self-analysis to recognize when we do this. It can interfere with your ability to relate to a health care worker and this, in turn, has a domino effect resulting in less care. Try to recognize this feeling if it occurs.

Of equal importance is the counter-transference ambush. In a war, the enemy may draw you into life threatening situations by deliberate traps and deceptive maneuvers. In a hospital, your caregivers may inadvertently damage you with the counter-transference trap. Counter-transference is the mental process by which a person transfers feelings from important figures in his or her life onto clients. It is often defined as the caregiver's feelings about the patient.

Uncle Tony

Over many years, I had the opportunity to listen to my husband, Joe, as he talked to patients over the phone. One of the perks or disadvantages of being married to a counselor, it depends on how you look at it, was that I was able to give him immediate feedback on his interactions. I usually rated him as a "B" or "B-". One evening as I listened, I was surprised to hear how annoyed he was and very abrupt, which wasn't his style with patients.

I asked him, "Joe, what's going on, you seem so annoyed." He replied, "I don't know, he really got to me, he sounded so like my Uncle Tony when he was complaining and finding fault." I responded, "You took your feelings toward your uncle and transferred them to your patient. I'm afraid I would have to give you a "D" on that interaction."

Caregivers are individuals with personal history, values and bias. Transference and counter-transference are processes that are always examined in psychiatric settings. They also apply to the nurse/patient, doctor/patient, and health care worker/patient relationships in hospitals. We need to talk about their presence in hospital relationships.

So what is one to do? Obviously, you can't undo the psychological underpinnings of your caregiver. But if you notice any of the following behaviors bring them up for discussion:
- Anger at you for the simplest request
- Avoidance behavior – present only when called
- No engagement in your effort to be involved in your care
- Blatant hostility or disrespect

Use these statements:

Patient: *I need your care but I get the feeling you're annoyed with me and I don't know why.*
Ideally, this gives the caregiver the opportunity to reply:
Nurse: *I didn't realize I was coming across that way. I'm so sorry, I had a very bad week and I shouldn't take it out on you.*
Or

*I can't believe it. I'm talking to you like I
talk to my Aunt Mary.*

But we don't live in an ideal world. If you get more hostility and
the response is more anger, it is time now to ask the nurse manager for
a new caregiver.

Patient: *It seems that you're not happy caring for
me and that makes me very anxious and uncomfortable and I need another nurse. I would
like to speak with the nurse manager.*

If you do not get a positive response from the nurse manager, you
can go up the chain of command and ask to speak to the supervisor.
You may choose to say nothing but be aware that it will impact on the
quality of your care. We'll look at another example of staff anger later
in our clinical tale "Epidural Nightmare".

Bias in Hospital Care

A March 2002 *Institute of Medicine* report found that racial and
ethnic minorities receive lower quality health care than whites. In a
2004 report released by the U.S. Department of Health and Human
Services, it was reported that black women had less thorough care than
white women based on 69 quality measures. A further example, the
University of California reported that with patients who came in with
broken arms and legs, only half of Hispanic patients were given pain
medication, compared with 75 percent of whites. These are only three
of multiple studies that point to a very serious health care issue, bias
in health care delivery. It is a very complex problem that extends to
bedside care. What should the minority patient or any patient who is
different look for and do?

Justifiably, minority patients mistrust medical and hospital care.
The causes and solutions for this serious health care issue are beyond
the scope of this book. But the manifestations of it at the hospital bed-

side need to be examined with bias exposed. Bias leads to avoidance behavior by staff and lower quality care and it cannot be ignored.

We are a multicultural society. The problem is, not all heath care workers are prepared to interact with diverse patients with sensitivity and respect for different cultures. If you are different by race, ethnic beliefs, lifestyle or behavior, you will be treated differently. It may not be obvious and often will be denied by the worker.

I wasn't sure how to include this section. The following story is not clinical but it impacted greatly on my view of empathy and caring.

Zeldia

As a member of a very liberal doctoral program in the '70s, we often had group sessions to expand our self-awareness. In one group session, a woman, in our discussion on prejudice, said "I know you you feel" to the only African-American woman in the group, Zeldia (I'll always remember her name). Zeldia replied, "Don't you dare say you know what I feel! Have you ever been in a room where you know "white folks" won't touch you because your skin is black? You have no idea how prejudice feels."

I remember thinking thank God I wasn't the one who said that and, more importantly, she's right. As a white, Irish, Catholic woman, I have no idea what prejudice is like. So right now I feel presumptuous in discussing racial and ethnic bias. No, that's not the word, I'm afraid I'll be insensitive in my "cultural sensitivity." What right do I have to recommend actions, yet I know that bias harms patients and impacts on quality care.

The fact is that patients are often treated differently in hospitals because of race, culture, lifestyle, or physical characteristics. It results in avoidance behavior by health care workers and directly impacts on your health care and survival. I can only stand witness and Zeldia, I hope I do it right.

If you asked any health care worker, including doctors and nurses, they would vehemently deny that any bias or prejudice enters into their care. They've been told from the beginning of their training that they have to treat every patient equally as a part of their professional role.

But my question is how many have looked at their own values and bias and checked to see if they influence the care they gave in any way?

Expressed, up-front examples of prejudice can be challenged but it is the insidious, unrecognized prejudices that are brought to health care that needs to be examined. One class on cultural sensitivity is not enough. No one likes to recognize bias exists in many health care workers.

The question is what can be done if your caregivers are not sensitive to your cultural needs? Your life and well being, as you know, are in their hands. You need to be alert to any racial or ethnic bias in the health care system. Health care professionals are now more diverse and registered nurses in particular have courses and workshops on cultural diversity in health and illness. Lack of cultural sensitivity and bias will result in less visibility and presence by the health care worker, avoidance of individuals and situations that make them uncomfortable. The basic ordered care will be done, but that will be it. Remember the patient at the end of the hall. You deserve more than that.

This issue involves not only cultural minorities but also any patient who is different. One group that is often discriminated against is the obese. No one would admit it, but judgments are made about lack of self-control, "They brought it on themselves." Jokes are made and staff may prefer not to care for obese patients. Another group that receives less care is the mentally ill. Untrained personnel are often fearful of the patient with a history of mental illness and the staff will often avoid them on a medical-surgical floor.

All patients and families need to be aware of quality of care issues. Patients who are minorities or have different lifestyles and values need to be doubly alert to incidents of diminished care. What can be done in a world of bias and stereotypes? How can culturally different patients make the hospital safer and more responsive to them?

Your knowledge of the hospital system and its culture can only help you to assess your care. It's difficult not to be mistrustful of all health care workers. Be watchful and identify a staff ally with whom you can discuss your concerns and figure out your actions. Confrontation, at this time of vulnerability, may be dangerous but reassignment of staff may be in your best interest.

Remember you have the right as a patient to request a different caregiver, one whom you can trust.

Bring bias into the discussion:

- *I get the feeling you're uncomfortable caring for me, is it because you're not familiar with my nationality?*

- *I know my size can be a lot to handle, how have you factored it into my nursing diagnosis?*

- *My wife has a long history of psychiatric care, I get the feeling that the staff are uncomfortable caring for her.*

Remember you are not accusing anyone of bias, you're just asking them to look at behavior that is impacting on you or a family member and the quality care you or they deserve.

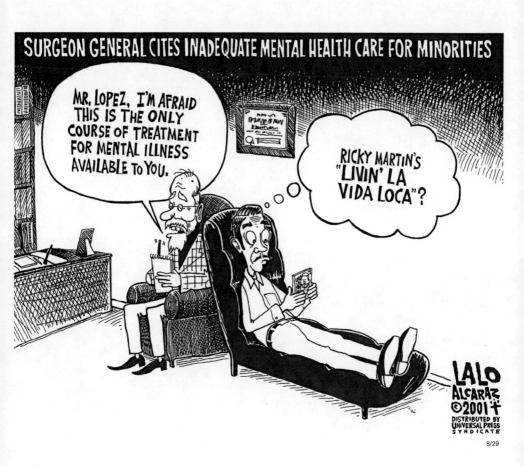

STRATEGIES FOR SUCCESS

After reading about the psychological dimensions of the battle, one may decide, "I'll just be the best patient I can, undemanding and everyone will like me." Not a good plan!

Miss Congeniality

Many years ago, when I was young and foolish, I tried the good patient plan during hospitalization for back surgery. I didn't want the staff to label me as a doctor's wife, as some prima donna who thinks she deserves special treatment. In my ongoing effort to be "Miss Congeniality", I never admitted my need for both physical and emotional care: Didn't use the call light, didn't ask for pain medication, and certainly didn't let them know I was scared!

While it was a successful operation, it was a terrible experience, made worse by my desire to be the good patient. After one week of bed rest, I inadvertently knocked the bedpan off the bed and urine spattered all over the room, the ultimate embarrassment. A nurse came in and cleaned it up as I was sobbing quietly. Notice the quiet. She never recognized me or my tears and, good patient that I was, I never said anything, suffered in silence as "good patients" do.

Obviously, I don't want you to use this plan. I was the "good patient" and probably everyone liked me, but I didn't get the care I needed, therefore, I was not successful. I got out alive but there could have been complications. There was a psychological cost, and I did not tell them about physical changes. Never again!

The following strategies will help you be a successful patient in your battle plan:

- Be a team member and be respectful of caregivers' expertise.

- Ask questions not as a critic, but to be involved in personal care.

- Be vigilant for non-verbal communication by the health care worker that impact on your care.

- Recognize personal needs, both physical and psychological, and ask for help.

- Focus anger on illness, not displacing it onto caregivers.

- Recognize vulnerability but not helplessness.

- Possess a knowledge base that allows dialogue with the caregiver.

- Don't let avoidance behavior by the staff, for whatever the reason, cheat you out of quality care.

- Recognize situations that call for assertive action and proceed to demand quality care.

- Don't hesitate to go up the chain of command when necessary. If you have serious concerns about the life of your family member, and the staff does not respond in a timely manner, call professionals outside the hospital to get results.

- Be alert for non-verbal examples of staff bias.

SURPRISE ATTACKS

Emergency Room

Emergency rooms are not a place you want to be but they can save you or your family member's life. Pre-planning should include an ER battle plan. You never know when your grandson, Gregory, will jump on your futon at camp, split open his forehead, and require stitches. You have researched in advance the site of the battle including the emergency room closest to home, and frequent out-of-town shopping and vacation sites. Questions to ask as you survey facilities:

- *Do you have emergency room physicians who specialize in emergency care?*

- *Do interns and residents staff your emergency room?*

- *How many registered nurses are working on each shift?*

- *Do you have two sections in your ER; one for emergencies and one for non-acute care?*

101

- *Can I stay with my family member when they are being examined and treated? (You will not be able to stay in acute life-threatening situations)*

- *What is your policy if I need to be admitted and there are no hospital beds free? Do I stay in the Emergency Room?*

- *When do you contact my primary physician?*

- *Do you have specialists on call: cardiologists, neurologists, orthopedists, hospitalists, and plastic surgeons?*

- *Do you have a special stroke protocol?*

When you go to an emergency room, expect to wait. Some authors have suggested going in an ambulance so you will be seen quickly. The ethics of this are questionable and the triage nurse will recognize the ploy. Tying up an ambulance that is needed to save a life should not be contemplated.

Of life-saving importance, you should use an ambulance for chest pain, signs of a stroke, major bleeding, or any other serious conditions. Trying to walk to the emergency room or use your own car can be deadly in those instances. Time is crucial!

In the ER, you should plan to use this time constructively and lessen stress:

- Bring comfort objects for children such as a blanket, toy, or hand-held computer game. Adults also need comforting - religious books, rosaries, or a soft afghan.

- Have books, laptops and video games to pass the time. Ask a family member to be responsible for their security. Staring at the TV and fellow patients can be anxiety producing.

- Begin conversations with fellow families in the waiting room if they seem receptive. Pass the time and also find out more about the ER.

- Avoid sitting next to someone that is obviously coughing and has a respiratory illness. The staff should isolate him from other patients.

- Don't hesitate to notify the staff if you see any change in your family member's condition.

- Don't attack the staff for the delays. Instead, ask:

I know how busy you are. Can you give me an idea of when my grandson will be seen?

- Remember that the number of acute, life-threatening cases drives the pace of the ER. If you are not one of them, be thankful. If you are, you must have immediate care and the triage nurse will see that it occurs.

- Don't try to use connections, "My friend is CEO of this hospital." or "My husband works for Senator..." Professionals who are trained to respond according to seriousness of the illness are offended if you imply connections give privilege.

- Try to avoid emergency rooms as much as possible by following good health care measures and preventing accidents.

We've covered key psychological dimensions of your deployment to the hospital, the language of war, and the "minefields". Now we move to your knowledge base in order for you to assess and monitor the quality of care that you or your family member receives.

DEPLOYMENT
FIELD MANUAL NOTES

Personal Notes:

- *Questions to ask when and to whom, follow-up questions*
- *Your nursing diagnoses*
- *Medical words and abbreviations to question*
- *Emotions you and your family are feeling*
- *Negative emotions you are sensing from health care workers*

PART THREE

ENGAGEMENT

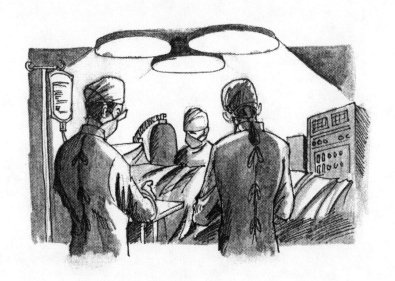

Voices:
Nurse and Doctor

SNEAK ATTACK – THE HIDDEN ENEMY

Enemy – Staphylococcus Aureus-MRSA

One may choose to worry about smallpox and anthrax but a germ that should be on everyone's radar screen is methicillin resistant staphylococcus aureus. Staphylococcus aureus is a bacterial infection that is further defined by the letters *MRSA*, the resistance to antibiotic therapy. The "terrorist attack" has already arrived on our shores. The National Center for Disease Control estimated 90,000 deaths in the year 2000 related to hospital infections. Nearly three-quarters of those deaths were preventable. **Deaths linked to hospital acquired infection (nosocomial infections) kill more individuals than breast cancer or car crashes.** Deaths are reported as statistics but these numbers do not reflect the thousands of individuals who survive but are forced to undergo additional extensive, painful surgical procedures and long-term antibiotic therapy. Some estimates cite as many as two million hospital patients may develop infections of varying severity each year. Where is the public outrage and concern? There are several groups that understand the problem and focus exclusively on hospital infections and are sources for information (www.HospitalInfection.com). Still, the great majority of individuals are not aware that hospital infections are life threatening and increasing in severity from year to year. We intend that this book is not only a wake-up call about hospital errors and infections but also contains strategies to fight them.

How can patients protect themselves in the hospital war zone? The first step in self-protection is an awareness that infections can and do happen. Hospitals are often viewed as ultra-clean, sterile environments, but in reality they are populated by human beings and bacteria that continually evolve and are extremely opportunistic. Hospitals, as any public facility, can harbor organisms in the tap water and even Legionnaire's Disease in the air conditioning system. You can't anticipate these, but you can control other pathogens you are exposed to in the hospital. Any break in procedure with a concurrent opening for bacteria, leads to infection. At the same time, the host (the hospital patient) is at their weakest point in health and resistance. It is a recipe for disaster and it is played out over and over again.

This field manual will describe step by step, the quality care that you should receive. These procedures are taught in Nursing 101 and if you know what to expect, you and your family can engage the health care worker in the on-going delivery of care that will win your battle against illness. Specific details give you power and questions that can be asked throughout the procedures help to ensure quality care and add redundancy to health care delivery. You are not assuming the role of critic, but rather one of learner since this is your body and life. Twenty years of teaching nursing are condensed into your engagement battle plan. The bibliography at the end was used to make sure no key points were forgotten. I visualize you, the reader, in a small classroom and I'm walking back and forth engaging you in your learning. The initial readers of the manuscript were the first class and their questions are reflected in your syllabus. Let's begin.

Hand Washing

Every book you read about hospital infections stresses the key element of proper hand washing by health care personnel. This is absolutely essential, but how do you as a patient know that they are doing it? On admission, ask the admitting nurse what the hand washing requirements are in this hospital.

- *Do they have specific sinks outside the rooms?*

- *Do the staff members wash their hands in the room bathrooms?*

- *How are doctors monitored for hand washing as they make their rounds?*

- *Does the hospital use antibacterial wipes plus hand washing between patient contacts?*

- *What methods do you use to keep the equipment used by all patients, for example, stethoscopes and blood pressure cuffs, from being a source of infection?*

As a part of your battle plan, you packed antibacterial wipes. You now ask staff and visitors to use the wipes before treatments or visiting. Have them use it on equipment including the stethoscope. A simple statement should be:

I know I may seem obsessive-compulsive about germs but all the stories I've read are scary. Please wipe off the stethoscope before you use it.

You're not implying that they don't use good hand washing technique, but the "I" message speaks to your vulnerability. A direct question to a caregiver, whether it's a doctor or nurse, is most appropriate. Then ask:

Did you wash your hands before coming in the room to do my care?

This type of question may make some caregivers defensive and they could lie to you, but you are putting them on notice that you are aware of their responsibility to prevent infection and that they must accept accountability. Observe how they respond to your question. Are they angry that you asked? Pick up on their anger:

You seem angry that I asked that question. I just want to be safe.

A true professional would respond positively to your question:
Thank you for reminding me, I know how frightening and serious infections are to you as a patient.

Reminders and accountability are your right. Don't let anyone intimidate you into giving up that right.

What You Need To Know Beyond Hand Washing

Most serious infections occur from invasive procedures that have compromised your skin barrier, your first line of defense. Dressing changes, wound irrigation, indwelling catheters, heparin wells, tracheotomies, and suction are all considered invasive procedures. The portal of entry of infection can be anywhere on the body including the skin, urinary tract, gastrointestinal tract, and respiratory tract. Let us examine specific procedure and your monitoring and engagement skills in this battle.

Dressings

Universal precautions is the proper disposal of hazardous wastes and was developed to protect the staff from getting infections from contaminated needles and body fluids and to protect patients and other individuals in the hospital from the spread of germs. One common misconception is the inappropriate use of the term "universal precautions". Individuals not familiar with the system may believe that if the staff is using universal precautions they, as patients, are protected from infection. Universal precautions offer protection, but only if the caregiver is concurrently using meticulous, sterile technique.

As a part of universal precautions, staff members are trained to:
- Place soiled dressings or used syringes into designated collection areas.
- Follow procedures for double bagging, labeling, and removal of contaminated items from the unit and hospital.

This does offer you protection from infection, but if the caregiver violates sterile procedure, infection will occur.

What do you need to watch for during a dressing change? What is sterile technique? Sterile technique is taking a sterilized dressing or instrument, one that is free from germs, and not contaminating it by touching non-sterile surfaces as you use it. It is also called aseptic technique, without sepsis, infection. This seems simple, but successful technique demands constant attention and vigilance. The staff can become blasé and careless with proper technique if they have done it for a long time and short cuts may seem attractive to save time.

Contamination happens and needs to be recognized as it occurs. The danger is with those caregivers who, for whatever reason, lack training or are in a hurry, contaminate a dressing or a catheter and don't recognize that they've done it. That is why a second pair of eyes, yours or a family member's are important – the redundancy equation.

You, as a patient, or a family member need to know the proper way that these procedures should be done so you can monitor the care that you or your family is receiving. You may have trouble looking at the incision and need to look away from the wound. If you know this about yourself, have someone there at dressing change time, preferably the person who will do the dressing change at home. It is difficult to look at a wound in your own body and some individuals can never do this. If you can, say to yourself:

This is my body and I need to know how it is healing and that the caregiver is doing the procedure in a way that will promote healing.

General Principles of Wound Healing

In order to monitor a dressing change, you need to know how it should be done correctly and how the body heals. When the skin integrity is broken, an infection can happen at any time, from a simple abrasion to a major injury. A large number of infections occur in the surgical units, where an intentional wound has been inflicted.

During surgery the edges of a surgical wound are placed adjacent to each other and the goal is to have the wound heal by primary intention, wounds that heal by secondary intention do not have the edges together. If the edges are not together, healing occurs by granulation from the bottom up. The initial blood clot holds the edges together and the body's defenses rush in to heal the break in its wall. Increased blood flow, white blood cells, fibroblasts, protein and building materials for granulation tissue are carried to the scene of the injury. If infection does not occur, collagen is formed and epithelial cells begin to develop. A scar may also develop.

Every procedure in wound care is designed to assist the process and not interfere with normal healing. That is one of the reasons why infection control is crucial. Often, a drain will be placed in a surgical wound and the reason for this is very simple. If too much fluid builds up in a wound, the edges of the wound will not join together and healing will be delayed or not occur. Fluid in the wound is also an excellent breeding ground for bacteria. Fluid comes out of a drain, but contamination can also go into a drain, so care of the drain is a very important dimension of wound care. Dressings may be either dry or moist depending on the preference of the surgeon. A moist dressing incorporates sterile, normal saline that may be heated if it is ordered. Questions to ask at this time would be:

- *Why do I have a moist dressing and not a dry one?*

- *What solution do you use?*

- *Since bacteria grow in a moist space, am I more likely to get an infection?*

In most hospitals, the surgeon does the first dressing change but it is a major responsibility of the nurse to monitor the initial dressing. She needs to check the dressing for intactness and for bleeding. There can be a small amount of drainage on the dressing and nurses are trained to circle it with a pen and monitor any increase. Patients with abdominal surgery need to be checked underneath their body because blood follows gravity and could pool under the patient. Family members should look at a dressing without touching it, note the amount of drainage, and also feel the bed linen under the patient to check for drainage. More than likely, everything is fine. But it is comforting to know that you are helping your family member in an important way.

Drain Care

If there is a drain, it will be attached to a suction machine or a small plastic container called a hemavac. The hemavac device is compressed, creating a vacuum, and as it expands the fluid is pulled out of the wound. The initial drainage will be bloody and this is normal. The quantity of the drainage is monitored and in the first post-op hours it is described as sanguineous drainage (bloody drainage). Over time, it should change to serosanguineous drainage and eventually to serous drainage (straw-colored fluid). It is well to note that only a few drops of blood make drainage or urine look bloody. Serious hemorrhaging is a different story and needs immediate attention.

As a family member, you can monitor the drainage. Change is of concern and should be reported to the nurse. For example, if the drainage becomes straw-colored and then bloody or increases in amount or stops altogether. Drains do become clogged and the sooner the drain is irrigated, the less damage occurs from backed-up fluid.

Orthopedic surgery is often very bloody particularly in the first 24 hours. The drain from a knee or hip is often attached to a device that collects the blood and it is given back to the patient as a transfusion. It is the patient's own blood that has been cleaned of debris by the micro filters of the device. If the patient and family understand the logic of the procedure, they can better monitor its use.

Evisceration/Dehiscence

In any surgery, but particularly in abdominal surgery, evisceration and dehiscence can occur. Evisceration is a fairly rare occurrence, and is found when the edges of the wound separate and the internal organs protrude, for example, the intestine through an abdominal wound. It is obviously a surgical emergency. Moist, sterile dressings are placed over the protrusion immediately and the patient returns to the operating room for repair. Dehiscence can be more common and it involves the separation and spreading of the wound edges. It indicates the wound is not healing by primary intention.

- Is there fluid buildup in the wound that has caused the separation?
- Has some stress such as coughing, lifting, unusual movements or simply going to the bathroom caused the separation?

Nurses know which individuals are at risk and an overweight patient or one who is compromised in healing, is prone to developing these complications. Splinting the wound with a pillow as you cough or go to the bathroom can help to lessen this occurrence. Proper wound healing is the goal of every soldier in the battle.

Dressing Change

What are the proper procedures that a nurse is taught and what appropriate, safe modifications can be made? The nurse will bring all the dressing materials into your room and begin to set up a sterile field. At no time should your old dressing be removed and the wound left unattended as the nurse runs out to get forgotten materials. The curtain is usually drawn for your privacy, but you have the right to have any family member there that you wish. As a family member, do not let them force you out of the room but stay out of the way at the head of the bed, holding your family member's hand. If the dressing change is extensive or painful, the nurse should offer pain medication 20 to 30 minutes before the dressing change. If it is not offered, you have the right to ask for it.

Sterile Dressing Procedure:

- Hand washing by the caregiver

- Sterile field set up - Paper with plastic placed on the bedside table in a manner whereby the topside remains sterile.

- Any sterile dressing materials such as 2x2's, 2x4's, instruments, basins, sterile syringes, if needed, are dropped onto the sterile field.

- Any packing material to be placed in the wound is removed from the bottle with sterile forceps, cut with sterile scissors and dropped on the sterile field.

- Anyone or any non-sterile material should not inadvertently touch the sterile field. Therefore, it should not be unattended after it is set up.

- Non-sterile gloves are used to remove the old dressing that is placed in an appropriate disposal bag. These gloves do not touch the wound.

- The amount and type of drainage on the old dressing and the condition of the wound, any odor, abnormal redness, swelling and stage of wound healing are noted and then recorded on the chart.

- Sterile gloves are put on in the approved manner, never contaminating them, and the caregiver begins to do the actual dressing.

- The wound may be cleansed with sterile normal saline or painted with Betadine, poured into the sterile basin on the sterile field before the sterile gloves are put on.

- If there is a drain, it is checked for patency, irrigated if necessary with sterile normal saline.

- Sterile gauze pads of various sizes (moist or dry) are placed on the wound with sterile gloves or forceps and then a larger, thicker abdominal pad is added on top.

- The dressing is secured by adhesive or Montgomery straps, which do not have to be removed at every dressing change.

- A binder, a cloth covering, may be added to give support to an abdominal wound.

This is the standard dressing technique and there will be variations depending on the site of the wound, but the key word is *sterile*, with no contamination.

A large sterile field is not used all the time; it depends on the complexity of the dressing change. A skilled nurse can open dressing packets without contaminating them and setting up several small sterile fields. But the basic concept remains - sterile gloves to place the sterile dressing, no contamination and proper technique. Discuss with the nurse how to maintain sterility and not contaminate since you will need to know this procedure at home. It reinforces the fact that you are knowledgeable and stimulates the nurses not to be careless. The staff should welcome interest and questions. Registered nurses are educators and can talk about what they are doing as they do the procedures because this is the dressing that a family member will need to monitor and change at home. You are not asking them to stop and teach you but rather to communicate to you as they do the procedure. A skilled professional will model correct technique and will not hesitate to acknowledge when they have broken technique and contaminated some part of the procedure.

Some questions you should ask as you participate in your own or your family member's dressing change are:

- *How does my wound look?*
- *Are there any signs of infection?*
- *Is it healing well?*
- *Why is it a moist dressing or dry dressing?*
- *How long will the drain be in place?*
- *Is it difficult to put on sterile gloves and not contaminate them?*
- *What will you write in the chart about my wound and dressing?*

Each hospital ward usually has their own procedure manual. They may have added new procedures and techniques, but they should all be based on sterile technique. All points I have listed are concepts that allow you to ask knowledgeable questions throughout the procedures. They may say:

We don't do it that way anymore.

Your response:

How does this procedure protect me more thoroughly from infection than the steps that I learned in my field manual?

Enemy - Clostridium Difficile

Clostridium difficile is a gastrointestinal pathogen that causes diarrhea and possible electrolyte imbalance if not treated aggressively. It is particularly dangerous for the elderly in nursing homes and hospitals because any patient in a weakened state is compromised by such an infection. In the June 2005 *Internal Medicine News*, it was reported that a new toxic clostridium difficile strain has been seen in nine states. It is an aggressive, more virulent nosocomial infection leading to graver complications. The need for prevention of this serious illness is crucial in preventing hospital deaths.

Isolation

Patients with this nosocomial infection will be cared for with some type of isolation precautions. The best defense is the rigorous hand washing by the staff and your awareness of the cleanliness of your personal space.

Have your family walk through the unit to observe isolation or enteric precaution signs. You are well protected from infection where strict isolation is in place since isolation is a very rigid and protective procedure where a known infection is kept from other patients and staff.

Obviously, the staff will not tell you what infection is present but an appropriate statement and question would be:

- My family has noted isolation signs, what additional precautions are you taking on the unit to insure no spread of the infection?

There should be additional emphasis on hand washing, use of gloves and disposal of waste products. If you or your family member gets this infection, treatment will probably include medication, but of equal importance is strict monitoring of intake and output.

- What measures are being taken to make sure my mother is getting enough fluids?

If you note that the patient in the other bed in your mother's room shows signs of bowel problems (frequent bedpans or bathroom trips), ask questions of the staff:

- I noticed Mrs. Wright seems to have some gastrointestinal problems, what are you doing extra to prevent possible spread of infection?

- Do you use isolation early with the initial signs of any bowel problem?

Feeding Tubes

One entry point for gastrointestinal (G.I.) infections are feeding tubes. These are often ordered for the elderly or for any medical condition that interferes with swallowing. Because the G.I. tract is not sterile, this is a clean procedure with hand washing and clean equipment. But infections do occur if the following rules are not followed:

- The solution used in continuous feedings should not hang for more than eight hours since microorganisms grow in warm environments.

- Feeding sets and tubing should be changed every 24 hours to protect the patient from the growth of microorganisms in the equipment. The times for changing the equipment should be clearly marked on the tubing.
- Every time the feeding is started, the tubing should be checked for correct placement in the G.I. tract to make sure it is not in the respiratory tract, trachea or lungs.

Ask the following questions:

- *What is the hospital's policy for how often they change feeding tubes and solutions?*

- *How do you check for correct placement of my mother's feeding tube?*

This is a reminder of your knowledge of correct procedures and your desire to understand your family member's care.

Enemy – Streptococcal Pneumonia

Any respiratory infection is dangerous for a hospitalized patient. Signs are often posted limiting visitors who have colds or flu. Grandma may really want to see the grandchildren but little ones are often reservoirs for various viruses and bacteria. You should screen your visitors and ask them to leave if they have any cold symptoms such as sneezing or coughing and say:

I appreciate you coming to see me, but if I catch a cold I'm in real trouble.

If they do not respond, the nurse may insist they leave or at the very least, wear a mask. Staff members should not come to work with any infection, including a respiratory one. If your caregiver has a cold, you have the right to request another one, or ask them to wear a mask. This includes your physician.

There are multiple organisms that can cause infections but we are using one as an example to give you principles and a focus for all infections in each system: skin, gastrointestinal, respiratory, and urinary. Respiratory infections range from "simple" colds to pneumonia and modes of entry can be procedures that involve tubes and breathing devices commonly used in hospitals; ventilators, tracheotomies and suctioning.

Assessment

Your first line of defense is monitoring and assessing your family member's respiration-rate, depth, any shortness of breath, cough, pain or any increase in sighing. It is very difficult to monitor your own respirations because once you bring it into consciousness, the tendency is to breathe differently. You can, however, notice change. As in any assessment, changes need to be reported and assessed. Vital signs will be checked including pulse, respiratory rate and blood pressure. The sooner a respiratory infection is diagnosed and usually verified with a sputum culture, appropriate treatment can begin.

The respiratory system is so closely associated with your heart and circulatory system that respiratory symptoms can often be the first sign of cardiac problems. Lack of oxygen (hypoxia) can be present with a variety of indications before vital signs change, and may be vague: restlessness, apprehension, anxiety, decreased ability to concentrate, increased fatigue, dizziness, behavioral changes. Other signs are more specific: pallor, cyanosis (blue color in hands and lips), and shortness of breath. You, as a family member, can be the first to note these signs and changes and they require immediate attention by the staff. Delay will not be acceptable.

Complex Procedures

There are also very complex procedures, for example, thoracentesis (removing fluid with a needle from the pleural sac), the use of artificial ventilating devices and chest tubes. Patients with these devices are often in the Intensive Care Unit. You won't be involved in the complex monitoring on this unit but you have a right to ask questions so you can be alert to any changes in your family member's condition. Don't let the setting intimidate you. You don't have to understand everything to ask the following questions:

- *What do you do to specifically insure sterile technique in such a complex procedure?*

- *Is my family member given any medication to help her tolerate this very difficult treatment?*

- *How is my family member's comfort monitored while on the ventilator or with the chest tube?*

- *What emergency procedures are in place if the electricity goes out?*

- *What if the tubing or chest drainage bottles become damaged?*

- *When you get a chance, would you explain to me how this device helps my family member?*

Asking "what if" questions are very important.

Pulse Oximetry – This sensor device measures oxygen saturation level in your blood and can monitor respiratory function. This is a fairly simple non-invasive procedure that shouldn't cause infection unless the caregiver coughs on you or scratches the skin on application. It is included in your field manual since it demonstrates the care that the nurse is taught to take, even in a fairly routine procedure. You, as a patient, should expect care in placement of the device so it is accurate and cannot cause impaired circulation or compression damage. It can be placed on a finger, ear lobe, toe or the bridge of the nose. The device will not work if it is attached to an inappropriate site. You will then observe the nurse:

- Check for capillary refill (pressing on the toe or finger to ascertain peripheral circulatory status).
- Read sensor levels frequently while giving care.
- Move sensors every four hours and spring-tension sensors every two hours.

Questions to ask:

- *How did you choose this site for the device?*
- *How frequently do you read the sensor levels?*
- *When do you move the sensor?*
- *What should I look for as I read the device?*

Discuss the sensor reading with the nurse so that you can do ongoing readings as a member of the care team. It is not difficult to understand normal ranges and you may, in fact, be the first to notice change. The nurse can reply, "This is well within the normal fluctuations of the sensor reading." Or, "That has definitely changed, I'll check your husband's vital signs and we'll keep a closer eye on it." Either response is reassuring and fosters an ongoing communication with the staff.

Suctioning

The next section of your field manual focuses on an invasive procedure called "suctioning". The patient will be encouraged by the nurse to cough, deep breath and use a spirometer (a device to measure effectiveness of breathing) to keep his airway open and bring up secretions.

While this can be painful post-surgery, it is crucial to prevent infection and promote recovery. Appropriate pain control is also helpful in order to allow the patient to cough and deep breath.

If one is not able to clear secretions orally or if a tracheotomy (surgical opening in the trachea) is in place, suctioning is performed to "clear the airway". It can be done through the back of the nose or mouth or deeper down into the trachea. There are a variety of oral airways and tracheal devices. Suctioning is a very uncomfortable procedure, not one a patient can monitor himself but one you, as a team member, need to understand and question. Organisms introduced into the trachea and lungs can cause major, serious infections.

Suctioning of the mouth and nose is considered a clean procedure but suctioning of the trachea requires sterile technique. Remember the steps in a dressing change. The same sterile technique is used: sterile gloves, sterile equipment and a sterile field. The need for suctioning is determined by proper assessment of each individual patient by inspection and use of a stethoscope. It is a traumatic procedure and shouldn't be routinely prescribed every one to two hours for all patients. Some may need it every hour, some every four hours.

Often, the suction devices (bottle and suction machine) are on the hospital wall and the age and size of the patient determines the proper suction pressure. Excessive negative suction pressure can damage the nasal and tracheal tissues and provide a site for infection. Some physicians and hospitals may require extra oxygen before suctioning but research findings vary on the need for this. It may be comforting to the patient to receive extra oxygen before suctioning if his diagnosis does not counter-indicate this.

A sterile drape is set on the patient's chest, a sterile catheter does not touch any non-sterile surface; sterile normal saline is placed in a sterile basin and sterile water-soluble lubricant is put on the catheter tip. Sterile, sterile, sterile! Often nurses will have a sterile glove on their dominant hand, which handles the catheter that is inserted, and a non-sterile glove on their non-dominant hand to connect tubing and regulate suctioning pressure.

The lubricated sterile catheter is inserted gently through the nose or mouth. The distance the tube is inserted depends on the size and age of the patient, and the catheter is inserted without suction. When in place, intermittent suction should be up to 10 seconds at a time. Oxygen does not reach the lungs during suctioning, so the patient needs to rest between the application of the suction. The tube is often rotated as it is removed and the patient may be instructed to move their head from right to left during the procedure.

You may not want to know all of this, but remember you are in a war, and respiratory infection kills. Hopefully, you can be there during the procedure, holding your family member's hand, standing at the head of the bed, asking questions and interacting with the caregiver. Questions to ask:

- *How do you maintain the sterility of the catheter?*

- *Should my husband have a little more oxygen or medication before the procedure?*

- *How far do you put the catheter in and how long do you leave the suction on?*

- *What if he starts gagging or is very uncomfortable?*

- *How often will you do the procedure and what should I look for to know when he needs suctioning?*

- *How do you monitor him after suctioning?*

This is a life-saving procedure, but not a pleasant one and the more you know the more you can be a part of the team to prevent infection. With some variations, the patient can be suctioned through an artificial airway such as a tracheotomy tube but the principles of sterility, proper amount of suction and timing need to be maintained.

Oxygen Administration

If your family member is receiving oxygen, there should be no smoking in the room; oxygen is a highly combustible gas. Hospitals are smoke-free, but you also need to be vigilant. If they are receiving oxygen it is often with a nasal cannula. Placement of the cannula is considered a clean procedure with proper hand washing. The rate and flow of the oxygen should be monitored and the condition of the nasal opening is checked for any breakdown. Here are some questions to ask:

- *What is the flow rate of oxygen and how is it determined by the doctor?*
- *What would be the signs that he isn't getting enough oxygen?*
- *How much water needs to be kept in the humidification bottle at all times?*
- *What type of solution do you use in the humidification bottle?*

The right solution must be used in the humidification bottle, where the oxygen bubbles through the liquid. It must be changed frequently per hospital policy. The solution is an environment conducive to the growth of bacteria and a source of nosocomial infections.

Enemy – Escherichia coli (E. coli)

You know how to protect yourself in dressing changes, respiratory therapies and ways to prevent gastrointestinal infections. Now we look at strategies to prevent urinary tract infections with proper urinary catheter care. There are many invasive, humiliating procedures that one must submit to in a hospital. Having your urine collected in a bag is one of them. It is also one of the prime sources of hospital-based infections. E. coli is a bowel bacterium; one of many that can cause urinary tract infections and the catheter is a primary source.

Catheters

Urinary catheters may be inserted in the operating room and are removed post-operatively when your output of urine is sufficient. Other catheters are indwelling and are left in for a longer period of time, for example, following prostate surgery or with an elderly, incontinent patient.

As a member of the team monitoring and assessing both you, as a patient, or as you assess a family member, one area that needs vigilance is intake and output (I&O). How much does one drink and eat compared to how much fluid goes out through urine, sweat or is lost through the gastrointestinal tract. The reason that this is so important is that the relationship between fluids and electrolytes, (those compounds that affect all the organs in our bodies including our hearts) is very delicate. Too much sodium and/or too little potassium can cause problems. Measuring urinary output is a key element in monitoring overall health status, and families are encouraged to share in keeping track of intake and output. You can be the first to note that your mother is not drinking much or that the urine in her catheter bag seems darker than usual. Concentrated urine and lack of intake fluids needs to be assessed and actions taken immediately.

If the catheter is inserted on the unit and not in the operating room, sterile procedures need to be followed to the letter. There are intermittent catheterization procedures and indwelling catheters with a balloon anchor, inserted in the bladder. Catheters have different diameters and are ordered depending on the patient's needs. Catheters can be a major source for urinary infection and should not be used unless absolutely necessary.

It was at this point, that I almost lost a reader, my son, Tom. "I don't really want to learn about balloon catheters." Hopefully, Tom, you won't need to know this but if in the future you do, you can refer back to this field manual. I don't expect any reader to remember all of the details. I recommend, as you read, jot down questions that you can ask your nurse. The field manual is the basis for knowledgeable, specific questions that you can ask as needed. Tom kept on reading as a "good son" and had helpful questions for the book.

Insertion of a Catheter

Obviously, it's difficult to watch yourself being catheterized but the questions and observations should be ongoing. This is not a time for modesty, remember this is a battle for survival, so if there are family members present have them observe from the head of the bed. The family member is the cognitive, interactive voice for proper aseptic (without infection) technique. The key elements of proper procedure include:

- Expect the nurse to explain the procedure to you and your family and get extra help if your family member is disoriented. It is important to have sufficient lighting to do the procedure properly.

- A bath blanket should be draped over the patient to preserve modesty.

- Disposable gloves will be applied and the area washed with soap and water.

- A sterile catheterization kit will be used.

- Sterile gloves will be applied to arrange equipment on the sterile field: catheter, lubricant, the sterile water and syringe for an indwelling catheter, cotton balls with antiseptic solution, sterile drape.

- After a sterile drape is carefully placed, the nurse will cleanse the area with antiseptic solution using the dominant hand and forceps. The non-dominant hand has opened up the area around the opening.

- The nurse will pick up the catheter with the dominant, sterile hand, coiling the catheter in the palm and inserting the lubricated catheter tip into the opening.

- The patient will be asked to relax and take a deep breath, and the catheter should not be forced if resistance is met during the procedure.

- A urine specimen is collected in a sterile container if ordered; the bladder is emptied and the balloon is inflated if it is an indwelling catheter.

Why do I include all this detail? The procedure requires step-by-step care to insure sterile technique and you, as the patient, should expect this scrupulous care. It is not a procedure a nurse should do in a quick, careless manner. Expert nurses can do it efficiently and well but they should not skip steps. These are some questions to ask:

- *Is it hard to handle all the equipment in a sterile manner?*

- *What does it mean to use the dominant or non-dominant hand?*

- *How often will I need to have this done?*

- *My mother now has an indwelling catheter in place, is she more apt to get an infection?*

- *How often will the indwelling catheter be changed and do you irrigate it?*

- *Does the urine that you were able to obtain look concentrated or bloody?*

- *Do you have procedures to keep the private areas clean to prevent infections?*

- *Do I need to do anything to make sure the indwelling catheter is draining well?*

- *Can I walk around with my catheter bag?*

- *Should my mother drink more since she has an indwelling catheter?*

- *What do I do if the tubing to the collection bag becomes unattached?*

Answers to Questions:

Private areas should be cleansed twice a day if an indwelling catheter is in place. The caregiver should always have the catheter bag below the level of the bladder in bed and during transportation to prevent ascending bacteria. If the bag is raised in transportation to a stretcher, the tubing should be clamped. Check to see there are no kinks in the tubing and the amount of urine in the collection bag is increasing.

As you walk, the bag needs to be lower than your bladder. Patients in wheelchairs can have the drainage bags placed in a more inconspicuous covering. If permitted by the patient's condition and doctor's orders, intake of fluids for a patient with an indwelling catheter will be 2000 to 2500 ml. a day.

A closed system is never disconnected. Urine is emptied from the drainage port every 8 hours or sooner if needed. If the tubing becomes unattached, the ends of the tubing should be wiped with antiseptic solution before reattaching.

As always, these questions focus on involving you and your family in your care and in this case preventing urinary tract infections.

Cornered

by Mike Baldwin

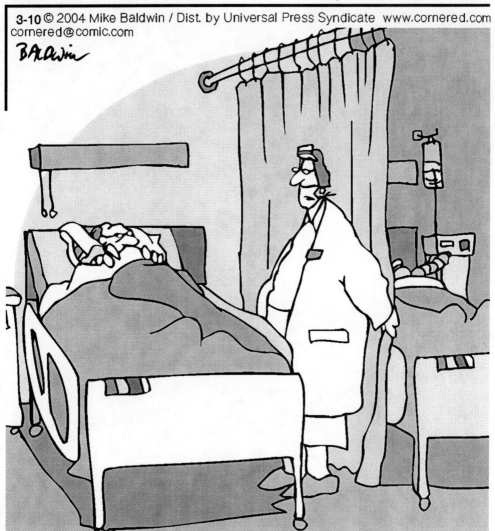

3-10 © 2004 Mike Baldwin / Dist. by Universal Press Syndicate www.cornered.com
cornered@comic.com

"The patient in the next bed is highly infectious. Thank God for these curtains."

PLANNED MANEUVERS – MEDICATION

Enemy: Adverse Drug Reactions

The administration of medications is to heal. Why then are medication errors in hospitals so widespread and life threatening? Medication errors are often categorized as iatrogenic injury - symptoms, ailments or disorders induced by drugs or surgery. Experts in hospital quality control have looked at doctor's handwriting, misuse of abbreviations, human error, lack of computerized technology, mathematical errors, misidentification of patients, and lack of training. Causation is complex. Some hospitals have banned certain abbreviations to reduce medication errors, and most hospitals have unit doses controlled by the hospital pharmacy and computerized systems to track medications. The recommendations to doctors include using the full words, not abbreviations, as examples,

- "Daily" instead of QD
- "Every other day" instead of QOD
- "Units" instead of IU or U
- Spell out "hours"
- Write "morphine", "magnesium sulfate", and "zinc sulfate"

Anything to reduce errors is valuable, but even new systems have drawbacks. Computerized systems have lessened errors but in some cases have contributed to new errors. How do you completely eliminate human error? As reported in <u>Internal Medicine World Report</u>, April 2005, the incorporation of computer technology seems to be a "double-edged sword". Information technology is still dependent on human input and health care personnel make mistakes. The health care system is trying to repair itself to eliminate errors, but change takes time and the basic premise of this book is that we, as patients, can't wait. We have to protect our families and ourselves. The best safety net for you and your family in the hospital is your knowledge and interaction in the process of medication administration and the principle of redundancy.

Let's start with your admission to the hospital. Every guide recommends that you have a list of your medications with you at all times, including dosage and frequency. But just handing it to the caregiver is not enough. It is a tool and the basis for all the medications you receive in the hospital. <u>The Archives of Internal Medicine</u>, February, 2005 reported that medication errors at the time of admission are common and some have the potential to cause harm. Medication errors can also occur when you are transferred to a new unit. Admission and transfers are key variables. Questions to ask:

- *There are many medications I take at home, has the doctor ordered them for me in the hospital?*

- *How do you make sure I have the same medications here in rehab as I had on 3 West?*

Some persistence with the questioning is necessary because there may be so many physicians involved in your care: an admitting MD, intern, resident, specialist and attending physician. Hopefully, they are all communicating, but you are the final expert on your care.

- *I always take Lipitor at home, is there a reason it wasn't ordered here in the hospital?*

- *I never took this pink pill before, is there a different type of Synthroid in the hospital?*

There can be a medically justified reason for change, but you have
a right to know it and your involvement is a part of your individual
safety net.

How is the nurse taught to administer medications ordered by the
physician? Your knowledge will allow you to check the process at every
level. She is taught to follow the five R's: <u>Right patient</u>, <u>Right medica-
tion</u>, <u>Right dosage</u>, <u>Right time</u> and <u>Right route</u>.

Right Patient

The nurse should say your name and check your armband before
she gives you the medication. Elderly patients can respond positively
to any name. After several days of administration of the same medication to you, she may just say your name but many nurses are trained
to continue checking the armband as a routine and safety check and
now many ask you for your birth date. If you have a very common last
name such as *Smith* or *Jones*, ask if there are anymore "Smiths" on the
unit. Staff should highlight this on the Kardex (cards that list each
individual patient's medication for each day) but your bringing it up is
appropriate.

- *I know in this area there are a lot of O'Briens,
are there anymore of us wandering around in this
unit?*

- *My mother gets so confused sometimes, she'd take
any medication anyone offered her. How do you
protect her from unordered medications?*

Right Medication

The nurse is trained to check the medication on the Kardex (there may be different names for this record of medications in different hospitals) and compare it to the doctor's orders. There are several medications that have similar generic names so she needs to check which one is ordered. Any new additional medication on the patient's Kardex needs to be checked with the doctor's order. This is where a patient or family member's questions are essential. The Kardex is on the medication cart or at the nurses' station and initialed by the nurse after she gives the medication. Ask to see it at least once during your hospital stay. You have a right to see it. She may say, "I'm too busy to show you now, I have so many medications to give, but I'll bring it in later and discuss it with you." It is important to bring the routine into individual perspective.

- *I have an extra pill today. What is it and why am I getting it?*

- *How do you spell that? I get very confused with all these medications, let me write it down.*

- *How do you keep track of all of my medications? Could I see the card you keep them on?*

- *Why is this initial circled or crossed out? (Indicates medication not given)*

- *Have you listed my allergies on the card?*

Right Dosage

This is a crucial element in medication administration and the nurse is trained to know the usual dosage for any medication and if it is a new order, she is taught to look it up in the drug manual in the ward. Errors are made with a simple decimal point. There is a big difference between 0.1 mgm and 1.0 mgm. Your questions should include:

- *Is this the usual dosage of this medication?*
- *How is it written, in milligrams? I always get confused with my math?*
- *Why am I getting more or less than the usual therapeutic dose?*
- *What is my mother's pulse rate?*
- *What is my blood pressure; prothrombin time/INR?*

This type of questioning is always important, but particularly critical when you are receiving a new medication. This is the time for you to learn and to become a second level of safety for yourself. Also, certain medications require the nurse to do checks before the medication is administered, including:

> ➢ Digitals – Apical pulse (stethoscope to the heart) to check to see if your pulse is above 60. If it is below 60, you don't get the medication.
> ➢ Blood Pressure Medication – Checking to see what your blood pressure reading is.
> ➢ Blood Thinning Medication – Checking to see what your prothrombin time/INR is.

Right Time

You've seen the abbreviations: Q.I.D. (four times a day), T.I.D. (three times a day) and Q.D. (daily). As we noted, many hospitals are reviewing these abbreviations and requiring doctors to eliminate them and spell their orders out. The time of medication administration is very important to maximize the drugs' effectiveness. The nurse learns to give the medication within one-half hour of the designated time: a medication ordered at 2:00 p.m. can be given from 1:30 to 2:30

p.m. Obviously, there must be some allowances for emergencies and the number of medications that need to be given to patients, but a 2:00 p.m. medication given at 3:30 p.m. needs an explanation. You're not attacking or being critical but a question is appropriate.

- *I know how busy everyone gets, but I didn't get my 2:00 p.m. medication until two hours later.*

- *I get worried when my mother gets her medication so much later than it was ordered.*

Some medications given later will not present a problem, but others are critical, heart medications, diuretics, and antibiotics to name a few. Your questions are all legitimate.

When you are awakened during the night to receive your antibiotic, it is important to know that antibiotics need to be given around the clock to maintain the proper blood level to fight infection; timing is crucial.

Right Route

Route designates the way the medication is delivered.
  PO – By mouth
  SL – Sublingual
  SC – Subcutaneous injection
  IM – Intramuscular injection
  IV – Intravenous administration

There can also be topical, intradermal, vaginal, instillations in the bladder and rectal administrations. Medications can be given by a variety of routes. Here the focus is on the most common and serious errors, but principles should be applied to any medication given by any route.

The key variable you need to be aware of is the speed with which the medication gets into your bloodstream, and if there is any safety margin for error. A patient can have a reaction to any medication given by any route but unless you are allergic to a particular medication (which is noted on your chart), taking the wrong medication by mouth can usually be remedied quickly as long as it is discovered in a timely manner. The body has ways to eliminate medications. Omission of required oral medication can be most damaging and your ongoing questions will help to prevent that occurrence. Remember medication errors can be both by commission or omission.

Sublingual, under the tongue medication, is absorbed very quickly as can be seen with nitroglycerin tablets given for angina - a specific medication with a specific route. Subcutaneous and intramuscular injections are absorbed more quickly than by mouth but less quickly than intravenously.

Injections

The angle of injection is important: 95 degrees intramuscular (IM), 45 degrees subcutaneous (SC), 15 degrees intradermal (I.D.), and of key importance and requiring particular care is the site of these injections. Each individual patient must be assessed for body fat, muscles and skin tone to give the injection with care. An elderly, frail woman may need a 15-degree angle and a short needle to get into muscle. Shots are routine, but they should never be given routinely. The right patient, medication, dosage, time and route all apply. There are strategies to lessen anxiety and pain – deep breathing, the position of the legs and toes (turning the toes inward if not contraindicated) and Z tract (pulling the subcutaneous tissue in a certain way). Ask the nurse:

- *I really get tense when I get a shot and it hurts. What can I do to relax?*
- *How do you pick the site where you give the shot?*
- *When my wife gives me my insulin shot, how should she figure out how and where to do it?*

Nurses spend a great deal of time learning where to give shots so as not to damage nerves: In the outer aspect of the deltoid (arm); upper quadrant of the dorsogluteal muscle (buttock), ventrogluteal (buttock); and the vastus lateralis (thigh). The site of the injection should be cleaned with antiseptic, the sterile needle put in at the correct angle and the syringe pulled back to see if the needle is in a blood vessel. If this happens a new injection site is chosen. The medication is injected and pressure is applied to the site after the needle is withdrawn. Routine yes, but it is an invasive procedure, and you need to make a point to ask questions about it. Remember registered nurses are educators and an ongoing discussion of technique can greatly enhance care.

Intravenous Therapy

In the intravenous route, the instant absorption of fluids or blood into the bloodstream needs particular attention and care. Medications and solutions introduced directly into the bloodstream have an immediate effect. There is no margin for error and the rules of <u>right patient</u>, <u>right route</u>, <u>right time</u>, <u>right medication</u> and <u>right dosage</u> are critical. Your attention, involvement and questions should be particularly focused on this (IV) route. You need to be involved in all your medications, but be particularly watchful with intravenous administrations.

Anything introduced into a vein must be sterile; all solutions, needles, over-the-needle plastic catheters, medications and PICC lines (peripherally inserted central catheters). Sterile techniques must be used in setting up the IV including inserting the needle into the vein or into the plastic catheter. Previously, if you needed an IV you had to be stuck every time with a needle, the catheter and rubber port eliminate this repeated, painful procedure. The site and the process of hanging subsequent IV's and mini-bags requires meticulous, sterile technique. You need to observe and question the following aspects of the procedure:

- Check on hand washing and ask when it was done.

- Question how and why the site was chosen for the IV: foot, hand, inner aspect of the elbow, or a central venous line?

Is it based on accessibility, not over joints or bony prominences or restricting the dominant hand and arm?

- Tubing should be inserted in the IV bag or bottle with a sterile spike and the infusion tubing will be filled with the solution to remove any air.

- The nurse will use clean gloves and cleanse the skin with an antiseptic before insertion into the patient. A sterile needle with or without a catheter is inserted into a vein. Many hospitals have IV teams who are particularly skilled in inserting IV's. If your nurse or technician has any trouble getting in the vein, going for more than two insertions, request another staff member.

I get so nervous with needles, I know you're trying but I need someone to get in right away.

- The nurse should check to see if the needle is in the vein by the blood return into the tubing or syringe. Some solutions, including chemotherapy, can be very damaging to tissue if the solution is infiltrating outside the vein.

- Two pieces of narrow tape are placed around the catheter and over the needle hub to keep it in place, a transparent dressing is applied over the IV site: the date, time, size of needle and initials of the nurse or technician should be attached to the dressing.

- The nurse should carefully adjust the flow rate (drops per minute) and continually monitor and assess the patient's response to the IV.

There are various intravenous solutions, for example, normal saline, 5 percent Dextrose and water, 10 percent Dextrose and water, and Ringers Solution, each ordered by the physician. As important as the right solution is, the amount you receive over 24 hours, and the drops per minute need to be calculated with care. Infusion pumps often regulate rate and flow but machines need to be programmed and monitored by nurses. When the machine beeps or buzzes have the nurse check it. Mini-bags, 50 cc as compared to 1000 cc IV bags are commonly used to deliver antibiotics. These can often be piggybacked with a larger IV (both hung at once at different heights, only one flows at a time). Questions you need to ask during insertion and subsequent care include:

- *How many liters of fluid have been ordered and how does that translate into drops per minute?*

- *If the IV stops flowing, what will you do to get it started again?*

- *What should I look for at the IV site to check for infection (redness, swelling, pain) and phlebitis (heat and/or redness over the path of a vein)?*

- *How often do you change the IV tubing (every 24 hours)? How often do you change the IV dressing (every 48 to 72 hours per hospital policy)?*

- *Are there any medications in my IV and why am I receiving them?*

Read the label and contents on the IV bag, you can touch it. After all, you're paying for it and it's your body. Never let a staff member really speed up the flow of an IV to make up time and deficit in IV infusion. Too much fluid, too quickly, can cause fluid overload in the circulatory system, especially in the elderly, and can cause serious consequences, even death. Pediatric IV's include calibrated drip chambers as a safety device to prevent too much fluid going into a very tiny circulatory system. Remember that the sterility of the IV system must be maintained when changing solutions, tubing and dressings. Hand washing, disposable gloves, and never allowing the ends of the IV system, either the spike into the bag or the needle or catheter into the vein, to become contaminated. You, as a patient, or family member can observe this.

What do you do if you accidentally touch the end of the tubing to a non-sterile surface?

The answer must always be:

I get new tubing.

Blood Transfusions

Blood transfusions can be life saving, but they can pose a life-threatening risk. You must be typed and cross-matched to the blood that you will receive. We often know our blood type, for example, A positive, but there are other factors in blood that need to be matched. There are safety precautions in hospitals involving the delivery of blood, including the procedure that two nurses must both check the proper type and cross-match for each patient. Even with this example of redundancy, let's add another check, the patient or a family member.

I understand my blood type is A positive, I would also like to check the bag for my name and blood type.

If they won't let you, I would refuse to let them hang the blood on my family member or me.

As with all IVs, blood transfusions are sterile procedures: needles, tubing, solution (blood) and proper technique. Blood transfusions require large gauge catheters or needles because of the thickness of the blood, and the site should be primed with 0.970 normal saline. The same solution is used after the transfusion and it is hung with the blood on "Y" tubing. Any other IV solution can result in hemolysis (destruction of blood cells).

The nurse should remain with the patient for the first 15 minutes when transfusion reactions are at the highest risk, monitoring skin color and vital signs. Blood needs to be infused over at least a two-hour period; some patients with a low fluid tolerance require four hours. Reactions to blood transfusions range from immediate low blood pressure, shock, fever, chills, to skin rash. Delayed reactions, several days or weeks after the transfusion, can also occur. If there is a reaction, the nurse stops the transfusion immediately, starts the normal saline solution through a clean (no blood in it) IV line to keep the vein open, notifies the physician, and remains with the patient, monitoring vital signs every five minutes.

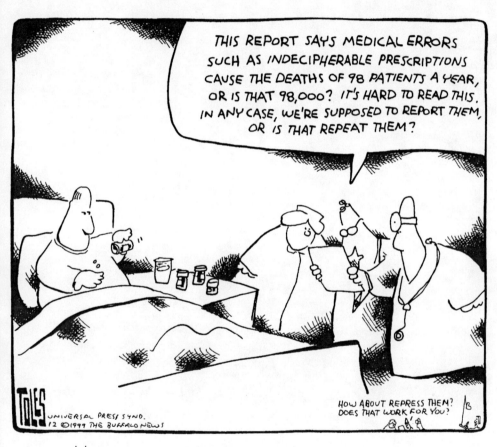

MOBILITY AS A DEFENSE AGAINST ATTACK

Enemy – Deep Vein Thrombosis (DVT)

You must keep on moving in a hospital for healing and to prevent complications. And you have to keep moving at a time when you or your family member feels weakest or is in pain. Every soldier knows that in a battle if he stays pinned in one position, the enemy knows where he is and the severity of attack can escalate. Calculated movement both protects him and allows for a better chance to counter attack.

In the hospital, your movement, in bed and ambulating, helps to protect you from your enemy, the deadly complication of deep vein thrombosis (DVT), a blood clot in one of your deep veins, usually in your leg. The life-threatening danger is that the clot can break off, travel to your lungs, and cause death from a venous thromboembolism (blood clot primarily to the lungs). Patients and families need to be proactive about the amount of activity you have in the hospital and at home. Get up and move as soon as your doctor allows it. If the doctor orders bed rest, ask him the reason for it and how long you will be bed-ridden. If you are on bed rest you will probably be on a blood thinner, have elastic stockings or IPC devices (intermittent pneumatic compression) ordered with some program of range of motion (ROM) exercises. If they are not ordered while on bed rest, ask why not.

I know immobility is dangerous, should I have some medication or devices to prevent DVT's?

Those of you who have had or will have orthopedic surgery, hip or knee surgery, will become familiar with continuous passive range of motion machines (CPM) that mechanically keep your limbs moving. These promote healing, flexibility and help prevent DVT's. DVT's can be deadly at any age with sustained immobility. What can you do to enhance your mobility?

- Cooperate with the nurse who is ordered to help you ambulate very quickly after surgery. Your first preference might be to just lay still, but lying there can be deadly.

- Ask to sit at the edge of the bed first before you get up, a safety measure to combat weakness and dizziness. Dangle your legs before you get up.

- Ask for a binder or support device before you get up if the surgical incision seems particularly painful.

- Don't get up the first time alone or just with a family member, have a nurse help you.

- Use a straight back chair as support for a few steps in the beginning.

- If you feel dizzy, tell the nurse and just sink down to the floor, as this is better than falling.

- Be insistent with the staff that if your family member can get out of bed, it be done on a regular basis. It's easier for the staff to make a bed if the patient is ambulatory or sitting in a chair.

- Monitor your or your family member's calves and thighs for pain, redness or swelling, report it to the nurse immediately. Pain may be the first sign of DVT, don't dismiss it as just muscle pain.

- Sitting for extended time in a wheelchair is still immobility. Even though you are out of bed it does not mean you are mobile. Positions need to be changed frequently.

Remember an active body will prevent complications and have a positive psychological effect on your recovery.

Bedsores

You may think that bedsores are just a problem in nursing homes. However, any confinement in one position for a long period of time can cause healthy skin to break down. On bed rest, mobility means turning to a new position at least every two hours. Bedsores are extremely difficult to treat for the elderly and it is of grave concern for a patient with diabetes. At any age, a break in the skin allows pathogens to enter and infection to begin, including the antibiotic resistant organisms. You need to get out of bed and move. Mobility is an excellent defense against your enemy, illness.

PAIN – ENEMY THAT ATTACKS RECOVERY

We've all experienced it, and basically it is the body's way of letting one know that there is damage, illness or limitation of function and it needs attention. Individuals who do not experience pain can do extreme damage to their bodies and not recognize illness. Pain is not something we choose and in the hospital it can impact on recovery, interfere with mobility, psychologically weaken us and become the enemy. It's difficult to fight disease, infection, and stay alert to quality care when you are in pain. It has been shown that pain is not always treated appropriately in hospitals.

Here are common misconceptions about pain:
- Minor illness causes less pain than severe conditions.
- Too much pain medication will lead to drug addiction.
- Caregivers can assess pain better than patients can.
- Some people exaggerate pain "It's all in their head."

Health professionals may try to respond to individuals in pain but they need help from patients in assessing the pain. Everyone has a different pain threshold and each caregiver needs to understand this crucial fact. Be clear in your own words about how the pain feels and don't let anyone dismiss your needs. Be persistent and have your team members be persistent.

- *I get the feeling you are not hearing me when I describe my pain. I need relief.*

- *I know everyone is different, but my pain is real.*

- *I understand that it's better to relieve pain early and not wait until it's excruciating.*

In <u>Internal Medicine World Report</u>, April 2003, several studies are cited that show physicians are "lazy" when it comes to pain management. It takes too much time to find out what multidisciplinary approaches can ease pain and it's easier to order a narcotic in the hospital. However, even though it is easier to order a drug, they still don't prescribe pain relief medication often enough. For many doctors, if they can't document a physical cause through test findings, they assume "it's not real pain". Not surprising, since doctors have received very little training in pain management in medical school. Nurses may also bring their own bias about pain to their patient care.

As the patient, you are the best judge of pain and should receive appropriate pain relief. Regular administration of pain medication has been shown to be more effective than delaying it until the patient is in agony. There are pain scales used by nurses to assess pain; namely location, severity, onset, duration, and aggravating factors. One can try to be stoic but pain relief will take more time and stronger doses may be needed the longer you wait to take it. Inform the nurse ahead of time that you will need pain medication to factor in any delay that arises from her other patients. Your team, spouse, and family members can also help you discover what comfort measures are helpful besides medication: change of position, back rub, food, heat or ice if ordered, music, picturing restful spaces, and distractions. Be particularly alert to pain in a new position in your body. You expect incisional pain but chest pain, arm or leg pain (any different site) should be brought immediately to the attention of the nurse.

If you are receiving pain medication, a diminished ability to monitor your own care can occur. This is the time to have team members with you at key points in your care, dressing changes, and new procedures. They may not be able to be with you all of the time, but help them figure out when they are needed.

Pain that is under treated has a domino effect on your recovery: less mobility, decreased appetite, decreased alertness to quality care, lower psychological strength; the possibility for DVT's, poor nutrition for healing, less involvement in care, and depression. Pain keeps you out of your major battle against illness.

Epidural Nightmare

Picture this:

Nancy, age 43, first pregnancy, six hours of labor on the obstetrics unit, four minutes apart, very strong contractions. She asked to have an epidural block, however, the nurse said it wasn't time yet. Nancy became more and more anxious and distraught. She begged for relief, finally her doctor was called and said keep her comfortable, give her the epidural. The nurses used their knowledge of labor, compared her to other women, and appeared to ignore her increasing anxiety and erratic heart rate on the monitor. Story ends there? No, now the nightmare begins.

The nurse anesthetist came into the room, obviously angry and unbelievably kicked the waste basket. She never introduced herself and promptly proceeded to lecture Nancy that it was too early, there are serious side effects, and listed all of the dire consequences. Remember, this is an extremely anxious woman and epidurals are given routinely in labor. The anesthetist seems to be punishing Nancy with graphic details for not following the staff nurse's advice. She would not let the husband stay, did the procedure, and stormed out of the room.

John, her husband, was afraid to say anything.

He thought he was going to explode in anger and he didn't want the epidural denied. What would you do? They were completely dependent, at 3:00 a.m., on one anesthetist. Her behavior was unprofessional and intolerable from any health care worker. Was she angry at the doctor for disagreeing with the nurses or upset because she had to get up at 3:00 a.m.? Who cares? She took it out on the patient, unacceptable! I question the safety of the procedure, a needle stuck in the spinal space by a nurse anesthetist who is angry and emotionally labile, a risk I wouldn't want to take.

What to do? Question the behavior first.

I don't understand, why are you so angry with my wife asking for pain relief?

I do not believe in this instance that would have helped because the nurse seems so out of control. Depending on her reply, the next statement should be:

I'm not comfortable, seeing you so angry, do the epidural for my wife. We need another anesthetist.

Probably, she'll say there's no one else at this time. Now is the time to go up the chain of command.

I need to talk to our doctor and call the Chief of Anesthesiology.

A letter of complaint will be sent to the hospital, outlining the incident and also questioning why the husband couldn't be with his anxious wife. Saying "that's the way it's done" is not acceptable to deny the husband's comforting presence.

I included this very recent clinical tale because it illustrates the lack of individualization in pain relief. This anxious patient needed help and her assessment of her pain level was discounted. However, of equal importance was the total unacceptable behavior of the nurse anesthetist. You use your "I messages" and team building skills but there are instances when you should demand better care using all the power you have. Don't let anyone intimidate you. Use the chain of command.

ENGAGEMENT
FIELD MANUAL NOTES

Personal Notes:
- *Allies' coverage and Roles*
- *Questions to ask when and to whom, follow-up questions - focus on procedures, medications and infection control.*
- *"What If" questions*
- *Telephone numbers of attending physician, health department emergency number.*
- *Record of severity of pain and response including medication.*
- *Record of mobility, times and activity.*

_____

_____

_____

_____

_____

_____

_____

_____

_____

_____

_____

PART FOUR

BEING SHIPPED HOME

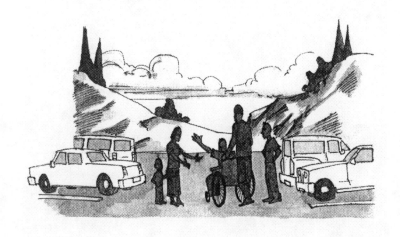

Voices:
Doctor and Mediator

EXIT STRATEGIES – DISCHARGE PLANNING

Weapons Needed

Discharge planning should begin on admission and your active participation in care puts you at an advantage for discharge. Much of the information that needs to be taught to you as you go home has been a part of your on-going involvement. You understand the standards of professional care: the steps in a sterile dressing, the procedures for medications and IV's, and the use of any equipment, for example: passive range of motion machines, oxygen, or suction devices. These standards will need to be followed in both the hospital and home.

It can be frightening being sent home, but hospital stays have been shortened considerably, and that in itself is not a bad thing. One fact is that nurses and doctors, as patients, want to be discharged as soon as possible. The less time spent in a hospital, the less chance for errors, complications or infection.

The summary of care in this book has allowed you to monitor, assess and be involved in your hospitalization. This book will not be sufficient instruction for you or your family members to do procedures at home. As part of a discharge plan, you should be taught hands-on instructions on how to do procedures and care at home. Your knowledge of the general principles of assessment, sterile technique and evaluating results will provide you with a strong basis to learn from the experts in the hospital and allow you to be an active participant in your recovery at home.

You, as a patient, should expect an interdisciplinary planning agenda that involves all your caregivers: social workers, dietitians, physical therapists, physicians and primary care nurses so that all dimensions of home health care are addressed. Hospitals, from both a humane and a realistic financial framework, have to do thorough discharge planning and teaching. Don't settle for a ten-minute, quick review of a sheet of paper, particularly if you have some complex care that needs to be continued at home. You want to be successful in your home health battle.

Questions to Ask

Put together with your allies a list of questions that you have developed throughout your hospitalization so that prior to the upcoming discharge you're ready. Specific questions should be:

- *Do I have enough support persons at home to aid in my recovery?*

- *Have you written a referral to a home health care agency? Why did you choose that agency?*

- *Will I have all my equipment I need when I get to my home?*

- *How will I be able to control pain?*

- *What level of physical activity will I be allowed?*

- *Do I get my newly ordered medications from the hospital pharmacy?*

You have already read your insurance policy but reimbursement for home health care is specific, very complex and always changing. Get what you need to continue the battle and then appeal insurance denial decisions if need be. We will go into detail concerning the appeal process later in this book.

Make sure the company you choose for your durable medical equipment (DME) - beds, commodes, oxygen equipment and disposable supplies is reimbursable through government or private insurance. Check your policy to see what is covered at home and for how long. Questions to ask both the insurance company and the medical equipment company:

- *How much coverage am I allowed for medical devices? What is the dollar figure?*

- *Is there a time limit on usage? When do I notify you to pick it up, days or a week before end of coverage?*

John's Hip

Doctors and providers of medical equipment for post-hospital use may use the following statement: "Of course you're covered." That is not enough proof of coverage. Read your policy again and ask for details from the insurance company.

Our son-in-law, John, didn't. His operation for a labial tear in the cartilage of his hip went well and he needed a CPM machine at home. He used it faithfully for four weeks and then called the company to pick it up and they came two weeks later. He found out the insurance company only would pay $1,500 and the rest ($1,400) was the family's responsibility.

A major shock and proof that the doctor's assurance and the device company's lack of up-front details proved costly. A week or two delay in picking up the equipment, deliberate or inadvertently, adds to the financial burden. This sticker shock could have been prevented by appropriate questions initially. They should have asked Mom and Dad.

Remember some policies do cover everything, some do not. What are the specifics in your policy? We recommended you check this out in the planning phase.

- *Does my policy cover physical therapy, skilled nursing care, medications and equipment?*

You're not going to get physical therapy to improve your golf swing, unless you were a professional golfer before your injury. Care at home is less costly for the insurance company than hospital stays so their financial goal will be to get you out as soon as possible. You need to get home also but you must be sure all of your emotional, physical, and financial supports are in place. Battles are often lost for lack of resources. Remember you are still in a battle against your illness.

Home Health Care

Check the credentials, accreditation and track record of any private home health agencies. The County Public Health nursing services and the Visiting Nurses' Association are strictly regulated for quality. In other home health agencies there may not be as much control of the care delivered in the home as there was in the hospital.

You and your family need to request registered nurses for skilled nursing care or highly qualified health care workers who have been trained and certified in home health care. All health care workers should be supervised by registered nurses and the care you exercised in choosing your hospital should extend to your home health care staff.

All discharge planning is crucial but certain health circumstances may require particular attention to detail and creative problem solving, for example, complex surgery and procedures, complicated pain control, and limited social supports.

Be diligent in selecting and assessing home health care. Use the same questions you used in the hospital to understand this crucial care. Do not accept lower standards on procedures. Sterile technique is sterile technique, whether in the hospital or at home.

Re-deployment to the War Zone

You've made it through your hospitalization, not only alive but also free of complications. Your battle plan worked but the enemy is strong. The illness has returned and you have to go back to the hospital, the site of your initial battle against the illness. Not only are you disappointed but also fearful that this illness is going to win. It is harder to fight a second battle against the old enemy, or maybe a new enemy that has joined the war.

Good soldiers rally, keep focused on the battle plan, and make adjustments for combat as needed and most important evaluate what happened so that it won't happen again.

- *Rally your support - spouse, children and friends. They're all disappointed you have to go back but they might have insights into the problem.*

- *Examine systematically the possible reasons for re-admission:*

- Not sufficient weapons to use at home.
- Personal depletion of energy beyond what is necessary for a successful recovery.
- Exposure to new pathogens.
- Errors made by home caregivers.
- Strengthening of the enemy, the illness.
- Need for re-treatment that can't be given in an alternate setting (not a hospital), for example, additional surgery.
- Sent home too soon.

The key to successful re-admission is to avoid labeling it as a failure on your part. You fought a good battle; some circumstances are beyond your control. It's now time to set a new battle plan in motion to defeat the enemy a second time! Get your team together, involve yourself in your treatments, assess, observe and be vigilant. You will get out of that hospital again as soon as possible with a new, realistic discharge plan based on what you learned the last time.

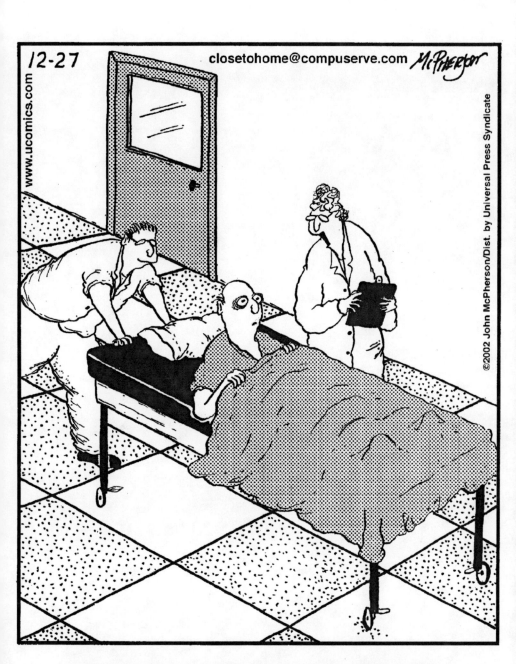

"We found out that your insurance was canceled three months ago, so we have to put your appendix back in."

INSURANCE COMPANY SKIRMISHES

Ally to Adversary

You may never need this section if everything goes smoothly and the insurance company pays the expenses and the pieces fall into place. Many readers of this book may not have health insurance, sad to say, as so many individuals and families do not. However, you will need to know how to negotiate with hospitals, doctors and possibly government programs. The strategies presented here can be used for any health care skirmish, now or in the future. Insurance companies are such major players in health care that to not discuss them would be to ignore the elephant in the living room. Here is the insurance elephant.

The following section starts with some philosophical observations about insurance companies and then presents strategies to deal with them. For this book it was necessary to look at the whole insurance industry and then use inductive reasoning, working from the broad concepts to specific processes, to simplify this complex subject. It hasn't been easy, but we will clarify some insurance company issues for you, with strategic responses.

When we listed your insurance company as an ally in your battle plan, we may have lost you. What were we thinking? The insurance company ally role can be defined as the checks and balances that this system provides by questioning and asking for accountability and documentation of quality care. Unnecessary procedures and extended hospitalization are not in your best interest and they drive up the cost of health care for everyone. Allies can change roles in the aftermath of battle and can drop out for a variety of reasons. Your view of the insurance company will change if there is a conflict over payment but remember the rules of engagement that we used during your hospitalization:

- Understand the characteristics of your foe, his strengths and weaknesses, and his vulnerable points.

- Approach any confrontation, whether by phone or mail, in a reasonable, unemotional manner.

- Don't get caught in the physician's battle with the insurance company.

- Never forget your real enemy is the illness. Don't deplete your energy in this ongoing negotiation with your insurance company. Get yourself better and then tackle this battle.

- Make sure your formal appeal is in letter form.

- Use your support allies to devise strategies and coordinate efforts.

- Be sure to follow up telephone calls with a letter stating the points covered.

- Keep copies of all e-mails.

The focus of this section is to outline facts and observations and devise strategies to maximize your efforts. Remember your ongoing goal has been to defeat the illness enemy. If you approach the insurance company in your attack mode, whether by phone, letter or in person, the company will in turn assume a defensive posture and the chances of a positive outcome for you will diminish.

Bottom Line

It is interesting to note that we seldom challenge an automobile or homeowner's policy with such comments as, "I know my deductible is $500, but given the circumstances of the accident, I feel I should only pay $250." Or, "I only have $30,000 in my homeowner's policy for household belongings but because of inflation they're now worth $50,000. I believe you should cover it." Insurance companies don't function that way, and you in fact have a contract in place with your company that stipulates limitations in coverage. Health insurance follows the same rules.

What are those health care businesses, who are the major players in decision making and how can I use insider knowledge of procedures, policies and personnel to get them to pay after the hospitalization? You read your policy before you went into the hospital. Read it again if you need to begin the appeals process, look for any ambiguity in definitions and terms. Read the appeals process and ask questions of the insurance company.

Let's look at the characteristics and make-up of health insurance companies. The bottom line of most insurance companies is to make a profit by controlling costs. In a certain sense, everyone should be concerned about health care costs. Businesses can't afford the expense; millions are uninsured and jobs are not being created.

The goal of keeping down costs seems reasonable to you, but not at your expense. You still want to have free choice, longer hospital stays, and all the procedures your doctor recommends. What can you do? As we stated before, and it is a key point, don't let yourself be dragged into the doctor's battle with the insurance company. Many doctors view insurance companies with anger and, you could argue, with good reason.

But his anger or mistrust does not have to be yours. The questions you need to ask are:

- *Why won't the insurance company pay for extended coverage?*

- *What can my doctor and hospital do to justify this need?*

Your doctor will make a strong case for the necessity of procedures or extended stay. An ethical doctor, however, will not lie to an insurance company to insure coverage is offered. Can he also make a strong case to the insurance company? If not, could there be some other reason for it not being covered?

Key facts that you need to know about your coverage when planning an appeal are:

- *Are physicians involved in making denial decisions?*

- *Who are they and what are their qualifications?*

- *Are they of the same specialty as your doctor?*

- *When do they come into the decision-making process?*

- *What are the qualifications and training of the registered nurses who often make preliminary decisions?*

You don't want these key decisions to be made by someone with no medical expertise.

Key Players

If the insurance company is viewed as your ally, then you can proceed to use the personnel and system to your best advantage. You don't go to Las Vegas without knowing the system. The Vegas system is to make money. The insurance system is to save money, and the best way to do that is to keep you healthy and get you well as soon as possible during hospitalization. Extended hospital stays due to infections and complications are not good for business. In summary, some key characteristics of health insurance companies are:

- Generally, a for-profit system: To save money for distribution to shareholders.

- Are regulated by state and federal statutes to provide health care dollars to policyholders.

- A key segment of health insurance company personnel consists of registered nurses and doctors who are by their professional license committed to quality patient care.

- There is an on-going tension and adversarial mode between doctors and health insurance companies.

- Accountability and checks and balances in health care can be used to your advantage.

- Medical directors are under pressure by their companies to keep costs down, but their professional license demands that they always focus on quality patient care.

Payment of costs is always a major concern for any family who has experienced a hospitalization. You read your policy in the planning stage and made the appropriate telephone calls in the deployment phase. Now you are home and the insurance company will not pay for all of your hospitalization. What can you do? You followed the doctor's recommendations for length of stay, tests and consultations, as you should. You asked appropriate questions throughout your care to understand what was ordered and why. You have read your appeals process in your insurance policy and have set the wheels in motion. You can scream and yell at the insurance company and even use the inside line that your doctor provided to yell at the medical director. This may be very satisfying but not an effective approach. The truth is that there is very little that you yourself can do in this phase except understand the process and make sure both the hospital and doctor are providing the insurance company with all the proper information and data. It is a business decision based on data, as are all business decisions. We'd all like to think that we are special and that our medical condition is unique, but in this phase we are more of a statistic. If you understand how decisions are made, and at what steps you can ask questions, it will add to the possible success of your appeal.

The one word you need to remember in this stage is <u>persistence</u>. Follow the process through to the final appeal and make sure you are clear that it cannot go any further. Is there an arbitration or mediation clause in your policy? You can always consider litigation but you need to know your chances of success, possible attorney fees and state regulations.

We recommend in this phase that you select one member of your team to be responsible for this ongoing process. The patient needs to continue the battle against the enemy, their illness, and does not need to be burdened with the demands and frustrations of appeal. Pick someone in your family who has a business background, is organized and likes to take on any system. This should be someone who can at least do the groundwork for you so that you can focus on your hospital discharge plan, your treatments, return visits to your MD, and on using your energy to get on with your life.

Your insurance company ally will be hindered somewhat by confidentiality regulations, in the sense that any direct contact with the insurance company will have to come from you, for example, letters and telephone calls. But behind the scenes your support personnel can collect general information, draft letters, and develop a list of questions to ask the insurance company, doctor or hospital.

Time Lines

Since both authors of this book would want to get out of any future hospitalization as quickly as possible, a re-reading of the coverage of our health policy was a necessity. Our policy has a Home Care Advocacy Program that requires pre-approval for paid-in-full benefits. The instructions require a doctor's prescription, a call even if Medicare is our primary insurance, and a list of what services are covered, including skilled nursing care, but not home health aides. Check your own policy for similarities or differences.

If the company decides that home health care, hospital days, treatments or surgery were not medically necessary or covered by the policy, instructions are provided for filing an appeal within a very specific timetable.

What the Hospital Needs to Do

Hospitals need to be paid in order to survive. In a certain sense the source of the payment is immaterial - government subsidies, insurance payments or private pay. Hospitals have therefore always been proactive in utilization review programs. Their CEO's and CFO's have been the pros in negotiating insurance payments but have not always been as forthright with information until after the bill is presented to the patient. In what other industry do you not get an estimate ahead of time before you contract for work? Their argument is that there are too many variables in hospitalization, but a listing of what will and will not be paid for by the insurance company is necessary to eliminate "sticker shock" at the end. Remember Andy Rooney's surprises.

What you want is fiscal accountability, no surprises at the end, and while the treatments and procedures are necessary, you need an explanation about how the hospital functions in relationship to Medicare, Medicaid and your insurance company.

The hospital usually gives you a discharge notice, which spells out your rights if you do not wish to be discharged. It includes telephone numbers to call and a specific time line. This type of notice plus other financial information should be given to you and your team before admission since that would be the time for your advocate to unravel and understand the fiscal dimensions of your care. After admission, your fight is to get well but your team can keep track of financial questions to ask the hospital. It does not help your recovery if you are burdened with surprise medical expenses after the fact.

The financial aspects of care are always changing. Hospitals used to be paid on a case-related basis, with so many days per condition. It appears that hospitals are returning to case rated or Diagnostic Related Groups (DRG) calculations, a flat fee for every admission, based on diagnosis. Sometimes it all seems like a game with the patient caught in the middle. But if the health care consumer knows the game plan, then appropriate questions can be asked of the hospital. The time line and rules may change for the battle, but the generals and majors in the hospitals, insurance companies, and doctors will try to financially out maneuver one other.

Where does that leave you? As my father would say, "Up a creek without a paddle." The proper questions at the right time can give you a paddle. The approaches to the delivery of compensation for the care of the patient is constantly changing and evolving beyond your control. However, questions that you ask before, during, and after your hospitalization can keep you in the loop and protect you from nasty surprises after the fact. Your before-hospitalization questions were included in your battle plan.

In Hospital

Here, your battle plan is focused on your enemy, the illness, and not on finances. But you or your advocate can ask a few simple questions of your doctor and the hospital's business office. The family does not want to be burdened with horrendous hospital bills after discharge:

- *My father seems better; can any of his care be done at home?*

- *Will there be any tests or procedures done over the weekend for my father?*

Many denial claims involve keeping patients with stable conditions in the hospital over the weekend when no tests or procedures are done.

After Hospitalization

Ask the insurance company, hospital and doctors:

- *After discharge, is all the equipment and nursing care covered by my insurance policy and for how long?*

- *What will you do (doctor or hospital) as part of an appeal to the insurance company if it is necessary?*

Remember, they may say everything is covered as in John's story, but you need to do your own homework about coverage. Questions bring the financial issues into discussion by all of the parties involved. They demonstrate that you and your team are knowledgeable consumers and emphasize the accountability of all of the participants in this complex issue of money. Be sure to check before hospitalization, what the hospital will do and what your rights are if the insurance company won't pay and check again in this skirmish:

- *Will they bill you for additional expenses? Does your contract hold the patient "harmless" for denied days?*

- *Do they bill you immediately and expect some payment?*

- *Are you liable for the bill during the appeal process?*

- *Are you or they responsible for the unpaid amount if the insurance appeal is not successful?*

- *What state laws protect you during and after this appeal time?*

- *How will it affect your credit rating if you allow the bill to remain unpaid during the appeal process or if you decide to not pay thereafter?*

Talk to representatives in the hospital's business office and your own financial advisor. Get straight answers and written policies before hospitalization. Be prepared. Keep excellent records. Try not to panic when you get that big bill; it is not good for your recovery. That's easier said than done, but remember it is a process and you and your team's persistence are key.

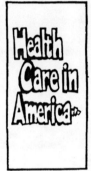

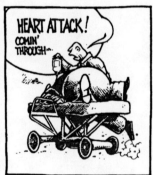

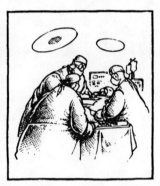

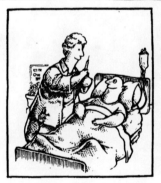

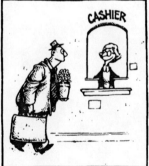

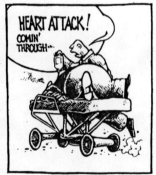

What the Doctor Needs to Do

Viewing your hospitalization from an insurance perspective, the doctor is the claims adjuster. He doesn't want to be, it has nothing to do with what he was trained to do, and he more than likely resents it. But he needs to be involved to get paid for his services. The insurance claims adjuster, whether an outside expert or an employee of the company, views the scene of the fire or accident and documents what damage has occurred, and the company bases payment on this assessment. The doctor needs to document the seriousness of your condition in progress notes based on his medical judgment so that payment of the claim is justified.

This seems straightforward, but when you are dealing with human beings, expectations of health care rights and the uncertainties of illness, it is very complicated. It often depends on the internal policies that the insurance company has, as well as the clinical expertise of the company's reviewers. However, there must be consistency and fairness in the decision, whether it's a president, cousin of a CEO in the insurance company, a friend of the governor, a clerk at General Electric or a construction worker on the N.Y.S. Thruway. Often, the initial claims personnel are not medically trained. What might be denied initially does not necessarily mean that it won't be subsequently covered by either grievance or appeal. Again we emphasize, follow the procedures through to the end, using all of the review services provided within the company and, if necessary, outside the company. Be persistent.

For the doctor, the rules have changed in the middle of the ball game, balls are not balls and strikes are not strikes, and the umpire (the insurance company) has taken over the game. A baseball metaphor seems most appropriate here.

Doctors have had many years of facing the reality of insurance companies. Wise physicians have accepted this reality and work toward helping their patients and ultimately themselves in getting financial support. Other doctors prefer to wage a war with the company and the medical director. It is regrettable that doctors often feel they have to kill the messenger, the insurance company nurse or medical director, when they are contacted about denials.

Doctor to Doctor Communications

Conversations with the attending physicians can be confrontational, educational and even humorous. I can remember a certain instance when one elderly surgeon told me in passing,"Sonny, why don't you get a real job."

Another physician practically cried on the phone and uttered, "I can't stand it anymore. I'm going to retire." I advised him not to, things would get better. I assumed a counselor's role and pointed out all the good things that he had done and will continue to do. One colleague on the phone wanted to know how I secured the job and asked if there were any openings for him!

A recent comment by the head of a department in a prestigious medical center did not help facilitate constructive dialogue. In a routine call to get more information on a patient and his condition, the doctor in a condescending tone demanded to know to whom he was speaking. The medical director identified herself and the doctor replied, "I thought I was speaking to a clerk pretending to be a doctor, now I know I'm talking to a doctor pretending to be a clerk." Despite this conversation, the case was decided on merit but confrontational rhetoric benefits no one.

What does the patient's physician need to do?

- Document completely the seriousness of the patient's condition, what clinical data supports this assessment and why these procedures are necessary.
- Treat the personnel, including RN's, at all levels in the system with respect, as this leads to discussion and a possible positive outcome. Channel their frustration with the system into posi-

tive actions that can bring about change in health care at the proper level, company and hospital or in the political arena.

What a Clinical Medical Director Does

A clinical medical director is a licensed physician usually in the state that the company is based. He is board certified in various specialties: family medicine, internal medicine, pediatrics or surgery and many have additional sub-specialty certification and credentials in such areas as geriatrics, pulmonary, or endocrinology.

The medical director for an HMO, my area of expertise, is responsible for reviews of utilization management cases (after initial review by trained utilization management nurses) when specific utilization guidelines are not met. These utilization guidelines include:

- *Initial pre-authorization* - As required by the specific contract

- *Extensions* - Continued case review

- *Retrospective case review* - Services which have already been delivered

- *Reconsideration review* - Whenever an adverse determination is rendered

- *Standard appeals review* - Routine appeals on a medical necessity denial

- *Expedited appeals review* - Appeals involving continued or extended services; additional services for members undergoing continued treatment. Any case in which a provider believes an immediate appeal is warranted.

The medical director uses corporate medical policy and nationally recognized standards as a guideline. The provider and the hospital or doctor are given the opportunity to discuss the clinical situation and the circumstances that require a specific action. However, what is usually required is actual office records or hospital charts to verify and justify the action taken.

My 16 years as a consultant and medical director for a large medical insurance company have given me a unique perspective on the system. Over the years I have developed a thick skin fielding attacks from my fellow physicians, some refusing to talk to me socially because of my role in utilization review and managed care. It has been my belief that patients come first and that each medical case is unique and should be treated as such. Guidelines are guidelines, but the individual patient and his response to the illness have not read these guidelines.

Most of the cases that are commonly reviewed now are the day-to-day evaluations of continued care in the hospital setting. As we stated earlier, the future will be that most hospitals will belong to case rated or DRG (Diagnosed Related Groups) settings, where the insurance company will try to prevent admissions if treatment could be done in an alternate setting. This will be to keep expenses down. The hospitals, however, will try to use medical necessity to justify admission, since they are reimbursed more for the admission. Some hospitals may even pressure doctors to admit patients to secure higher payment for the services. We shall see.

CAUCUS

The overall goal of this book has been to take the general concepts and distill them down to specific points, tools, skills, knowledge and questions. The health insurance section has been particularly difficult for me to focus on key points because of the ambiguous language, constant qualifiers and exceptions, insurance legalese and hidden agendas. How do you get a straight answer? We can assume your bottom line is "What do I have to pay?" Sometimes it seems too much. I'm sure the reader concurs.

My husband can describe and explain a physiological principle, a medical condition, or a treatment option in two or three clear, concise sentences. When he talks about the insurance process, he has adopted the company language, so I had to sit him down and ask specific questions, which helped me understand the system. I hope they help you. It had become very frustrating to me, a person who values simplicity in communication. I decided to use my skills as a mediator to highlight experiences and facts that you can use. I believe insider knowledge can only help in sorting out complex issues.

The following is one medical director's answers to specific questions. I believe that mediation serves a person well in situations where there are conflicting needs and agendas. Two of the major tools that a mediator uses are the ability to frame the issues and also use a caucus, private discussion with parties in a dispute to better understand the issues and plan future actions. I will try to frame the issues focusing on how one insurance company and one clinical medical director made decisions.

Q: *When do you get into the decision-making as medical director? How do you and the nurses collaborate in this process?*

A: After all the information is gathered and the nurse reviews the case, if she finds it does not meet the guidelines for intensity of service, the case is referred to the medical director. Rounds are made with the nurses daily to discuss case histories and particular guidelines are reviewed. Intensity of services and extenuating circumstances such as other conditions are discussed and a medical decision is made.

Q: *What does intensity of service mean and where do you get the guidelines?*

A: It refers to acute care that requires hospital admission or continuation of hospitalization. Nationally recognized guidelines have been developed by outside sources, which have determined standards of care, for example, both the Milliman organization and Medicare have well-established guidelines.

Q: *Let's focus on the hospital coverage decisions that are made while the patient is in the hospital.*

A: Medical necessity such as unstable vital signs, fever, severe pain, need for medical or surgical interventions that cannot be given outside the hospital determine continuation in a hospital setting. The key issue for continued health insurance coverage is whether the patient is stable and treatment could be given in an alternate setting, outside of the hospital setting.

Q: *Are practicing physicians aware of the guidelines for medical necessity?*

A: Source books, outlining what is covered and why, are provided to all physicians. Doctors should be aware of admission policies, standards of care, length of stay through both insurance company documents, and hospital utilization review policies.

Q: *Since you anticipate some anger from the attending doctors, how do you approach them with your questions?*

A: Many times the information I have received is minimal. I begin by saying, "Here is the information I have, help me out, what is really going on?" I often say, "Here's what I have. What would you do with this information; it doesn't meet any criteria, that's why I am denying it." Doctors are very busy and the MD's progress notes do not capture the true picture of the clinical condition.

Q: *Since you are not presently in clinical practice, how do you stay current in the clinical approaches and research?*

A: I attend weekly sub-specialty and grand rounds. The company provides a stipend for continuing education. I review multiple medical journals each month and I have access to the Internet to obtain up-to-date information on clinical practice. In addition, we have consultants in each specialty, and I frequently call local experts in each sub-specialty field concerning a particular issue around standards of care.

Q: *Give us an example of an in-house coverage decision and the key points you are looking for.*

A: A patient has had an acute heart attack. The guidelines specify a certain number of days of hospitalization. The nurse reviews the information from the hospital at the end of the allowed days. The patient's blood pressure is stable. There is no chest pain. He has been evaluated by various tests in the hospital. There has been no further surgery; after his cardiac catheterization (he may have had a stent or angioplasty) his heart rate is normal, there is no rhythm abnormality and he is up and walking without any problems or chest symptoms. There is no further evidence of a heart problem. The decision would be that a continued inpatient setting is no longer required. There are no other medical conditions that would require acute intervention.

Conversely, if any of the above conditions are not present, the hospital stay could be extended depending on his condition.

Q: *Where do you fit in with the post-hospitalization appeals process?*

A: I have a major role in the post-hospitalization appeals process. A different medical director from the one who made the initial determination, will review the case. This is the first level appeal. If it upholds the original determination of denial, a second level of appeal may be available. It will be spelled out in the contract. There is a difference between a grievance and an appeal.

Q: *What is the difference?*

A: A grievance has nothing to do with medical necessity, for example, it may involve medical equipment. An appeal examines medical necessity. Let me also define denial and medical necessity.

> ***Denial*** – the determination that the member does not have coverage for a requested or already delivered service or procedure. The denial may be based either on administrative or medical necessity grounds.

> ***Medical necessity*** - those criteria used to determine the appropriateness of the requested service and location of that service based on nationally recognized guidelines.

Q: *What are the major areas of appeal regarding hospitaliza-*
     tion and what key information would lead you to support
     the client's appeal submission?

A: The most common appeals are:

        - Prospective: A patient in the hospital challenges dis-
          charge.

        - Retrospective: After discharge for non-payment.

     After conversation with the attending physician, if he has
     described the patient's medical condition as not stable or safe
     for discharge, I would support the appeal. Examples: The pa-
     tient developed a temperature the night before discharge or de-
     veloped new symptoms (increasing abdominal pain, difficulty
     in breathing).

Q: *What key points would lead you to support the original de-*
     nial of coverage?

A: No new data that documents an unstable medical condition for
     continued inpatient setting would support the original denial.
     Post-hospitalization, many of the appeals are often surgeries
     that were considered cosmetic and not covered by the contract.
     They would be denied.

Q: *Have you been pressured by your insurance company to*
     deny claims?

A: The company does expect you to follow the guidelines to evalu-
     ate certain procedures. Every month there is a report generated
     to document the activities of each medical director. Each year
     the medical directors are monitored concerning compliance to
     internal guidelines. This is the reality of the system.

In my eleven years, I can honestly say that no one at any level of the company has ever said to me that my denial rate is too low. They respect my clinical expertise, and all of my decisions have been based on medical necessity and standards of quality care. The guidelines are only guidelines and there are multiple extenuating circumstances in which guidelines do not apply. I'm aware of the system, who wouldn't be, but I have never compromised my medical beliefs based on the system.

Q: *What do you believe hospitals need to do in denial of coverage cases?*

A: Hospitals need to submit the entire hospital record for review, not just piecemeal with a cover letter. We need doctors' progress notes, nurses' notes, medicine records, vital signs, operative notes. The entire chart, period.

Q: *What should physicians do in denial of coverage cases?*

A: Before the case is denied, the doctor should write complete and accurate progress notes. They are busy but this will ultimately save them time. The following one-sentence notes are not helpful:

> *"Patient doing well"*
> *"Clinically improved"*
> *"Probably will go home in a couple of days"*
> *"We'll discharge Monday"*

One excuse doctors often use is, *"I'm waiting for the test results."* Since they make A.M. rounds, they need to check the results in the afternoon to see if the hospital day is justified. Patients can be discharged in the afternoon or evening. By convention, the day doesn't count unless the patient stays beyond midnight. The day counts at midnight.

Q: *What advice would you give to discharged patients who are facing non-coverage bills?*

A: As usual, it depends on the contract; the hospital cannot bill you if you are a member of a health maintenance organization and the hospital participates. You may pay the deduction and some contracts have grace periods, if you stay an extra day, no matter what the circumstances, you don't have to pay. Check to see what your hospital does in your planning phase.

Patients need to know that there is a process called "reconsideration", whereby the medical director may get the denied case back if the hospital or attending physician submits new data pertinent to the case. Then there is an appeals process where an entirely different reviewer looks at the case. If the appeal is finally denied after review at all levels in the company, the patient may then have the option to go to an independent external appeal review. New York State has designated a process that, under NYS Public Health Law Article 49, provides an independent, external appeal review of the case through a Medical Care Ombudsman Program. Check your own state for external review programs.

Q: *Should the patient be pro-active in urging their physician to be diligent in their progress notes?*

A: (He smiles, thinking you poor, deluded woman) The patient is going to tell the doctor how to write his progress notes? Good luck!

Q: *How about a simple question during hospitalization such as, "What do you chart in my progress notes?" (to the doctor and nurses). At least you're letting them know that charting is important and that you and your team are paying attention.*

A: Remember that your financial insurance questions are for the planning stage and post-battle skirmishes. In the hospital, all your questions are asked to understand, monitor and assess your battle against the illness. The charting is the hospital and doctor's concern for quality care, reimbursement and malpractice issues. Save your questions during hospitalization to better understand your care, not to remind them of their responsibilities in charting.

One Final Note

Answers to these questions have been based on my work as a clinical medical director. I believe that these criteria should be met by all insurance clinical medical directors. Consistency and a uniform standard of professional practice would benefit the patient and enhance the credibility of the medical director with his physician colleagues. They probably will still not like the process, but the dialogue can be enhanced to benefit the patient.

The caucus is done, and I obtained permission to share it with the other parties, as all mediators do. Now it is time to frame the issues.

FRAMING THE ISSUES

This section about insurance was presented for your peace of mind. The first three sections: planning, deployment and engagement were developed to focus on your survival. It is important to concentrate on deployment and engagement while you are in the hospital as you monitor your care. Insurance cannot be ignored, no elephant can, but planning and insider knowledge can help you in your skirmish. It appears that the patient doesn't have as much control in this part of the battle plan as they may prefer. You have to depend on the doctors and hospital to present the data appropriately to the insurance company. After all, they want to be paid.

However, it would be wrong to imply that you do not have any control in the insurance skirmishes. You still have absolute control over your fight against the illness, rallying resources, monitoring care, conserving your energy to fight your primary foe, the illness. I would liken this phase to the negotiation process after a war, the treaty making, which is controlled by politicians. The politicians in this scenario are the doctors, hospitals and insurance companies. Personally, I like more control and I would have exercised my control efforts in the planning phase of the battle. Here, I know the process, who makes the decisions, and my rights. I also have a plan to conserve energy and let my advocates run interference for me. Well, I did finally get a football analogy in the book.

Armies and soldiers plan and strategize what battles to fight. They will not use their men and resources on unnecessary battles. The objective of winning the war is utmost in the soldiers' minds; therefore, some of the skirmishes need to be fought by allies. You need to prioritize the skirmishes and allow your allies, family advocates, and the hospitals and doctors to fight for reimbursement. Save your energy to get well. I know it is so distressing to hear from the doctor or hospital, "Your insurance company won't pay." But try not to get agitated even if the doctor or business office is implying you should be concerned. Stay cool!

Consider the following points and strategies:

- During hospitalization keep a log of the treatments, medications, and procedures you receive. Your advocate could keep this for you and the blank pages in this book will be your log. It's very difficult trying to remember after your hospital stay:

  - *Did I have IV's, go to X-ray, have blood drawn?*

  - *Did the doctor come in every day?*

  - *Who was that endocrinologist who saw me about my diabetes?*

It would be a good exercise for your anxious spouse or worried friend. Doing something in these situations gives one more of a sense of control. When that bill comes at the end of the hospitalization, you will have more personal data about what really happened. Keep all of your hospital bills, doctors' bills, and Medicare payments in a separate folder.

On receiving your bill, specific questions are appropriate if you have kept a record:

- *I believe my wife only received Intravenous therapy for 14 hours after surgery, the IV was pulled at 9:00 a.m.; the bill lists 15 IVs and four mini-bags.*

Errors happen in billing, hopefully inadvertently, but fiscal accountability can only be achieved with data. We're sure some readers will say, "I'm not going to be bothered doing that kind of record keeping." What we have tried to do is to give you multiple ideas for more control. Some will make much sense to you, others are not appropriate; pick and choose. Remember:

- You did your planning and you know what your policy covers from the specific questions you asked and recorded. You didn't let them hide in insurance language. Errors can be made in both coding the reimbursement request and billing.

- The initial reviewer may not have all the data or not understand the case.

- You have a long process of review, grievance or appeal.

- The doctor and hospital want to be paid and they have a whole hospital department or reimbursement system in their office in place.

- You know from pre-planning what your deductible is and if there are any fees that you will be responsible for, the bottom line.

- Some doctors may want to involve you in their reimbursement battle. You may choose to if you want to be involved, but remember energy lost here may take away from your recovery energy.

- There are outside processes beyond the insurance company you can utilize and persistence can pay off.

- Factor in the time and energy needed and how much money, out of pocket, you personally owe and develop a plan with your financial team.

These are post-battle skirmishes; the battle was fought in the hospital. You won that battle, you were discharged with no complications and you are on the road to recovery.

BEING SHIPPED HOME
FIELD MANUAL NOTES

Personal Notes:
- *Allies' roles*
- *Questions to ask when and to whom, follow-up questions*
- *Timelines of your policies' appeal process*
- *Telephone numbers of home health agency, equipment company, insurance company.*

_____

_____

_____

_____

_____

_____

_____

_____

_____

_____

_____

_____

_____

_____

END NOTE

This is the end of the class and book. I know we wandered a bit, but hopefully you followed along with us. I've never known an educator that doesn't do that on occasion, but the real art is guiding the student and the reader back to the key facts. We told you it wasn't a scholarly journey, but hopefully an interesting and practical one.

As we wrote in the introduction, two professionals have written this book, but it is not a professional book. My daughter suggested we "dumb it down", since she didn't want us to use "all of those high-sounding, educational and medical terms". Instead, we trusted in the intellect and common sense of our readers and tried not to drift off into "educationalese". It was hard not to use the word *collegial*.

This strategic field manual has been based on the "need to know" doctrine. The topics are complex, from procedures, psychological concepts, to insurance companies. The criteria for discussion have been simple explanations of complex subjects with specific realistic approaches. You have been given the tools to successfully transverse the minefields of health care. In any battle, winning comes down to utilization of your resources and a realistic appraisal of the situation. The hospital system is made up of human beings who are fallible, but who have also chosen this field in order to help those in need. Your active participation in the hospital experience can bring out the best in all caregivers and give you that extra energy and power to heal and survive. We can't change the world in one book, but we do want to initiate a process of bedside change in the hospital experience for patients and families. Delusions of grandeur, very likely, if no one reads the book. But it has been very satisfying to throw ideas out there, maybe no one will catch them, but isn't that what life is about?

The clinical tales have been the recounting of a professional journey; they are not major dramatic events, rather little pieces of life. They have always remained vivid in my memory. Why is it that certain interactions on our journeys are so memorable? I hope the sharing of these tales has been both interesting and thought-provoking.

I've included the last *Calvin and Hobbs* cartoon, which is not related to health care. However, it is my favorite because while I am realistic, I try to look with optimism to the future. It also allows me to use my second favorite word (after oxymoron), and that word is serendipity, a gift for finding good things unexpectedly.

We hope this book will help you and your family in your hospital experience. Get out of the hospital, healthy and stronger and continue on your life's journey.

End of Realistic, Philosophical Hospitalization 101.

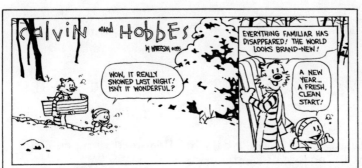

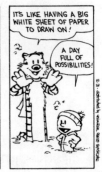

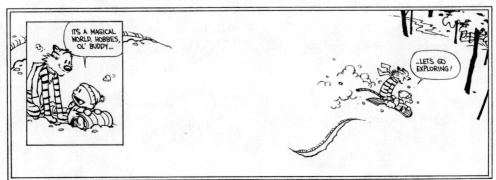

CITATIONS

Pen and Ink Drawings. Luke Santiago. Graphic Arts Student. Sage Colleges, Albany, NY. May 2005.

BIBLIOGRAPHY

Adams, Damon. "Minority Mistrust Still Haunts Medical Care." *American Medical News,* January 13 2003.

Bates, Betsy. "Toxic Clostridium Difficile Strain Seen in Nine States." *Internal Medicine News,* June 1 2005.

Cornish, Patricia et al. "Unintended Medication Discrepancies at the Time of Hospital Admission." *Archives of Internal Medicine*, February 28 2005.

DeLaune, Sue and Patricia Ladner. *Fundamentals of Nursing, Standards and Practice.* Albany, New York: Delmar Thompson Learning, 2002.

Ellis, Janice and Elizabeth Nowlis. *Nursing-A Human Needs Assessment.* Philadelphia: JB Lippincott Co., 1994.

Freiden, Joyce. "Pain Management-Physicians Too "Lazy" When it Comes to Pain Management." *Internal Medicine World Report,* April 2003.

Jaffer, Amir. "Preventing and Treating Thromboembolism in the 21st Century." *Cleveland Clinic Journal of Medicine*, April 2005.

Kohn, LT, JM Corrigan, and MS Donaldson (eds) and Committee on Quality of Health Care, Institute of Medicine. *To Err is Human: Building a Safer Health System.* Washington, DC: National Academy Press, 2000.

Krey, Mary Jo. *Management of Respiratory Infections: Practical Approaches.* <u>Cortlandt Forum</u>, April 2005.

Landrigan, Christopher et al. "Effect of Reducing Interns' Work Hours on Serious Medical Errors in Intensive Care Units." *New England Journal of Medicine,* October 28 2004.

Leape, Lucian and Donald Bewick. "Five Years after to Err is Human What Have We Learned?" *The Journal of the American Medical Association*. May 18 2005.

Lockley, Steven et al. "Effect of Reducing Interns' Weekly Work Hours on Sleep and Attentional Failures." *New England Journal of Medicine, October 28 2004*.

McVan, Barbara. *Illustrated Manual of Nursing Practice*. Springhouse Corporation. Springhouse, Pennsylvania, 1991.

Needleman, Jack, etal. "Nurse Staffing Levels and the Quality of Care in Hospitals." *New England Journal of Medicine*, May 30 2002.

Potter, Patricia Anne and Griffin Perry. *Fundamentals of Nursing Concepts, Process and Practice*. St. Louis, 2003.

Pope, Elizabeth. "Second Class Care." *AARP Bulletin*, November 2003.

Rundle, Rhonda. "Some Push to Make Hospitals Disclose Rates of Infection." *The Wall Street Journal*, February 1 2005.

Shannon, Margaret and Billie Wilson. *Drugs and Nursing Implications*. Appleton & Lange, 1992.

Siek, April and Louise Brenton. *The Nurse Communicates*. WB Sounders Company, 1997.

Taylor, Carol, Carol Lillis and Priscilla LeMone. *Fundamentals of Nursing: The Art and Science of Nursing Care*. Philadelphia: Lippincott-Raven, 1997.

INDEX

Printed in the United States
141866LV00003B/27/A